VICTORIA WILLS

DASH DIET COOKBOOK FOR BEGINNERS

The Complete 28-Day Dash Diet Meal Plan
+ 200 Flavorful Low-Salt Recipes to Lower Blood Pressure,
Gain Health Benefits, and Get in Shape Quickly

© Copyright 2020 - All rights reserved.

Table of Contents

Introduction

DASH stands for Dietary Approaches to Stop Hypertension. This type of diet is based on research carried out and funded on behalf of the US National Institute of Health (NIH). This research was about determining the role of diet on blood pressure. This diet was created to offer people who suffer from high blood pressure a delicious, tasty and balanced diet that lowers blood pressure at the same time. Therefore, this diet is primarily a diet to lower high blood pressure (more information on the DASH diet study in high blood pressure in the drug letter).

According to the NIH, the DASH diet promotes healthy eating habits. It offers healthy alternatives to junk food and processed foods. It aims to encourage people to reduce their salt consumption while increasing their calcium, magnesium, and potassium consumption.

Over the years, several other studies have proven the DASH diet is not only useful in lowering blood pressure, but that it is also useful in reducing the risk of cardiovascular disease, various cancers, stroke, diabetes, heart disease, kidney disease, heart failure and many more diseases.

The DASH diet is based on the following principles:

Reduction in salt consumption

One of the main goals of the DASH diet is to reduce the consumption of salt drastically.

Of course, man cannot live without salt. The human body contains around 150 to 300 grams of table salt. The amount of salt lost through sweating and other excretions must therefore be replaced. Salt supports the bone structure and digestion. It maintains the osmotic pressure in the vessels to keep the water and nutrient levels stable. But nowadays our foods are filled with too much salt - especially all processed products.

The extent to which increased salt consumption hurts health is currently the subject of intense discussion among experts, mainly since the body excretes excess salt.

But studies from 1970 in Finland already show that too much salt causes blood pressure to skyrocket. It could be demonstrated that reducing consumption of salt by 30% could even reduce mortality from heart attacks by 80%.

A study on mice published in 2007 at the University Hospital in Heidelberg showed that a lot of salt increases blood pressure: "Salt promotes the formation of certain messenger substances in the muscles of blood vessels that cause the muscle cells to contract. The increased resistance in the blood vessels increases blood pressure." The Heidelberg scientists therefore saw considerable advantages in reducing the amount of salt in food rather than prescribing conventional drugs.

There is disagreement among scientists about how high the maximum amount of salt should be. While US experts recommend a maximum of 1.5 grams of salt per day, the German Nutrition Society's recommendation is 6 grams per day and the upper limit is 10 grams per day. However, this only applies to a healthy person who moves sufficiently and is physically active and excretes the salt again through sweating. For example, an athlete can tolerate more salt than someone who only moves moderately.

I recommend that you only look at these values as a rough guide and gradually control your salt consumption as well as gradually reduce it. Also keep in mind that the maximum amount of salt you should consume depends on your body constitution and lifestyle.

Recommendation:

- Less is more! Therefore, pay more attention to your salt consumption in the future and reduce it step by step. The keyword is low-salt, but not salt-free!

- Avoid processed products (packaged food, pizza, French fries, chips, canned food, various meat and fish products, baked goods, etc.). If necessary, read the list of ingredients.

- If possible, use a natural salt substitute (herbs, etc.) in your meals

- Use low-water cooking methods such as stewing or steaming. This means the food remains tastier and you don't need to salt it as much (see also tips on reducing salt consumption).

More vitamin E and minerals

The DASH diet is based on a variety of fruits and vegetables and whole grain products to provide the body with plenty of vitamins and minerals. Particular attention is paid to minerals such as magnesium and potassium, which help lower or improve blood pressure.

More healthy fats and oils

Fats are energy carriers and ensure that fat-soluble vitamins such as vitamins E, D and K can be absorbed by the body at all. Certain fatty acids, such as omega-3 and omega-6 fatty acids, are also essential, which means we can only get them from food. Therefore, they should be on the regular meal plan. The omega-6/3 ratio plays a vital role in health. Omega-3 fatty acids help to maintain normal blood pressure levels wisely. However, our diet often contains too little omega-3 fatty acids. Good sources of this are fatty fish such as herring, mackerel, salmon, and sardines.

This also applies to the use of oils. Healthy oils include virgin cold-pressed olive oil and coconut oil (in organic quality versions). Unlike olive oil, coconut oil can also be heated and used for frying and baking. The much used sunflower oil, on the other hand, is less healthy because it only contains omega-6 fatty acids. This creates an imbalance in the omega-3 to omega-6 ratio. A ratio between 1: 2 and 1:5 should be aimed for.

Ultimately, as with most other diets, the DASH diet should avoid unhealthy fats, especially trans fats, a subgroup of unsaturated fatty acids, and replace them with healthy fats such as those found in nuts, seeds and fish. Trans fatty acids come from industrial production and are, for example, contained in chips, baked goods, French fries, confectionery, pizza, etc.

More fiber

Fiber is an integral part of the DASH diet. A fiber-rich diet, whether through fruits, vegetables, grains and cereals, has a positive effect on blood pressure and the cardiovascular system. (Evaluation of 24 publications between 1966-2003).

In contrast to the low carb diet, grain can therefore be consumed. However, it is essential to consume only wholesome grains (whole grain bread).

CHAPTER 1:

What Is The Dash Diet?

When the DASH study and the DASH sodium study were carried out more than two decades ago, it wasn't done to come up with a diet to promote weight loss. The researchers involved wanted to help hypertensive patients with a diet that also acted as an effective medicine. That being the case, weight reduction is presently the most famous aspect of this particular eating plan.

Companies and blogs who sell DASH inspired products often like to focus on the fact this diet will help you shed the extra pounds you've been battling to lose.

Not only will you be able to lose the unwanted pounds but, if you follow the diet with discipline, you will do so much faster than imagined.

And it shouldn't surprise you that the DASH diet can accomplish this. DASH is both a diet and a lifestyle. As such, you not only have to be mindful of what goes into your mouth. You are also expected to control how you conduct yourself.

DASH: The Diet

Three excellent factors make this eating plan great for those who want to look slimmer. Let's consider each of them.

Healthy fats

The first is that you are expected only to consume healthy fats. Good fats, as they are so often called.

You mustn't generalize and think all fats are bad for you. Even though it is a wide-spread belief that all fats will make it so you can no longer see your feet and endows you with a second chin, this isn't a fact.

The fats you should stay away from are trans-fat and saturated fat. All those scary things they have accused every type of fat of causing, trans and saturated fat are the actual culprits. Think about it: obesity, an increased risk of suffering hypertension and cancer, clogged arteries, and other kinds of heart disease. It's as a result of consuming those bad fats.

This doesn't mean that throwing caution to the wind and eating without any discipline doesn't play a role in causing these health conditions. But you greatly increase your risk by eating such artificial fats.

On the other hand, good fats are exactly what your body needs. These good or healthy fats include omega-3s and unsaturated fats. You know those times when you feel so tired, you can barely lift your hand as you lie in bed? Or the mornings you just get pissed at things that wouldn't matter to you on a good day? Your body very well may have been screaming for good fats.

Their many benefits including keeping your mind as sharp as a katana blade, giving you control over which way your mood should swing, helping you stay active all day, and promoting weight loss.

You read that right. Consuming unsaturated fats will help you lose those calories faster and healthier than if you try to do without them. Just as people get fats wrong, they also do the same with cholesterol. It has been so vilified at this point, that the mere mention of its name probably gives you heartburn. In reality, your entire body system would be thrown into chaos without cholesterol. The problem is when you consume too much of it. In life, if anything exceeds the bounds of moderation, then it is very likely dangerous. Your body also follows the same rule. Too little cholesterol and you might need to visit the doctor. Moderate cholesterol and your body will thank you for it. Too much cholesterol and you are making goo-goo eyes at the Grim Reaper.

To control your cholesterol levels, you should watch the fats you consume. Sticking with only healthy fats is a good way to make sure your cholesterol level stays moderate. And choosing the DASH diet is the overall best way to maintain a healthy intake of good fats.

High-fiber

Fiber is such an amazing nutrient; surprisingly, we don't eat it as often as we should. Most of the DASH diet foods are rich in both soluble and insoluble fibers, which is perfect for anyone dealing with digestive issues. Grains, fruits, vegetables, and legumes are some of the places where fiber is found in high quantities. If your grandma, or anyone else in your family, offered you some vegetables as a home remedy for constipation, then you've experienced one of the many benefits of consuming fiber. Did you know that the body can neither break down nor absorb fiber? It is unlike every other nutrient you take into your body. For example, fats are broken down into fatty acids and glycerol, and carbohydrates are broken down into glucose. Fibers just pass through your entire digestive system relatively unchanged. Again, fibers can be soluble or insoluble. This means they either dissolve in water or not. Soluble fibers, found in oats, apples, carrots, etc. are good for reducing cholesterol and glucose levels in the blood. Insoluble fibers, on the other hand, are helpful to individuals who are dealing with constipation. It also promotes stool bulk. You will find insoluble fibers in food sources like cauliflower and potatoes. While fibers absorb the water in your stool (Not something you want to read about? It'll be over soon) and make them bulky instead of loose, they also make them soft. As a result, your risk of getting hemorrhoids is reduced. Also, as common as diverticular disease is, you can avoid getting it. You may think it's no big deal, but you could suffer abdominal pain if those small pouches in your intestinal walls become inflamed.

Suppose that isn't incentive enough for you to start chowing down on some fruits, veggies, and legumes. In that case, you should know that a high-fiber diet helps lower your risk of colorectal cancer. Some scientists even believe that dietary fiber may be useful to prevent many colon diseases (Mayo Clinic, 2018). There is ongoing research to prove this. The deal-breaker for you could be this: switching to a high-fiber diet will prevent your blood sugar from spiking. As a result, and because your digestion has now been improved, fat will not be stored in your belly.

Benefits

The DASH diet comes with a range of health benefits. Following are some of the major advantages of following the DASH diet:

Cardiovascular Health

The DASH diet decreases your consumption of refined carbohydrates by increasing your consumption of foods high in potassium and dietary fiber (fruits, vegetables, and whole grains). In addition, it diminishes your consumption of saturated fats. Therefore, the DASH diet has a favorable effect on your lipid profile and glucose tolerance, which reduces the prevalence of metabolic syndrome (MS) in post-menopausal women.

Reports state that a diet limited to 500 calories favors a loss of 17% of total body weight in 6 months in overweight women. This reduces the prevalence of MS by 15%. However, when this diet follows the patterns of the DASH diet, while triglycerides decrease in a similar way, the reduction in weight and BP is even greater.

It also reduces blood sugar and increases HDL, which decreases the prevalence of MS in 35% of women. These results contrast with those of other studies, which have reported that the DASH diet alone, i.e., without caloric restriction, does not affect HDL and glycemia. This means that the effects of the DASH diet on MS are associated mainly with the greater reduction in BP and that, for more changes, the diet would be required to be combined with weight loss.

Helpful for Patients with Diabetes

The DASH diet has also been shown to help reduce inflammatory and coagulation factors (C-reactive protein and fibrinogen) in patients with diabetes. These benefits are associated with the contribution of antioxidants and fibers, given the high consumption of fruits and vegetables that the DASH diet requires. In addition, the DASH diet has been shown to reduce total cholesterol and LDL, which reduces the estimated 10-year cardiovascular risk.

Epidemiological studies have determined that women in the highest quintile of food consumption according to the DASH diet have a 24% to 33% lower risk of coronary events and an 18% lower risk of a cerebrovascular event. Similarly, a meta-analysis of six observational studies has determined that the DASH diet can reduce the risk of cardiovascular events by 20%.

Weight Reduction

Limited research associates the DASH diet, in isolation, with weight reduction. In some studies, weight reduction was greater when the subject was on the DASH diet as compared to an isocaloric controlled diet. This could be related to the higher calcium intake and lower energy density of the DASH diet. The American guidelines for the treatment of obesity emphasize that, regardless of diet, a caloric restriction would be the most important factor in reducing weight.

However, several studies have made an association between (1) greater weight and fat loss in diets and (2) caloric restriction and higher calcium intake. Studies have also observed an inverse association between dairy consumption and body mass index (BMI). In obese patients, weight loss has been reported as being 170% higher after 24 weeks on a hypocaloric diet with high calcium intake.

In addition, the loss of trunk fat was reported to be 34% of the total weight loss as compared to only 21% in a control diet. It has also been determined that a calcium intake of 20 mg per gram has a protective effect in overweight middle-aged women. This would be equivalent to 1,275 mg of calcium for a western diet of 1,700 kcal. It has been suggested that low calcium intake increases the circulating level of the parathyroid hormone and vitamin D, which have been shown to increase the level of cytosolic calcium in adipocytes in vitro, changing the metabolism of lipolysis to lipogenesis.

Despite these reports, the effect that diet-provided calcium has on women's weight after menopause is a controversial subject. An epidemiological study has noted that a sedentary lifestyle and, to a lesser extent, caloric intake are associated with post-menopausal weight gain, though calcium intake is not associated with it. The average calcium intake in this group of women is approximately 1,000 mg, which would be low. Another study of post-menopausal women shows that calcium and vitamin D supplementation in those with a calcium intake of less than 1,200 mg per day decreases the risk of weight gain by 11%.

In short, the DASH diet is favorable, both in weight control and in the regulation of fatty tissue deposits, due to its high calcium content (1,200 mg/day). The contribution of calcium apparently plays a vital role in the regulation of lipogenesis.

Just a little break to ask you something that means a lot to me:

What Did You Think of Dash Diet Cookbook for Beginners?

First of all, thank you for purchasing this book **Dash Diet Cookbook for Beginners**. I know you could have picked between a significant number of cookbooks, but you chose this one, and for that, I am incredibly grateful.

I hope it will add value and quality to your everyday life. If it were so, it would be nice if you could share this book with your friends and family by posting on Facebook and Twitter.

If you enjoyed this book and found some benefit in reading this, I'd like to hear from you and hope that you could take some time to post a review on Amazon. Your feedback and support will significantly improve my writing craft for future projects and make this cookbook even better.

If you have purchased the paperback version through Amazon, just going to your purchases section and Click "Write a Review", or if you have purchased it in a library, just going to Amazon and search this book (Title and the Name of the Author) and click "Write a Review".

I want you to know that your review is very important, I will be happy to hear your thoughts about this cookbook.

I wish you all the best in your future success!

Victoria Wills

CHAPTER 2:

What To Eat And Avoid?

What To Eat

- Plenty of fresh vegetables, especially lots of greens - almost without restriction
- Fresh fruit
- Lean meats, especially white meat (chicken, turkey)
- Whole grain / whole grain products
- Fish
- Protein-rich foods
- Foods with unsaturated and healthy fats such as nuts and avocados
- Healthy oils with an optimal Omega 3 / 6 ratio such as olive oil and coconut oil
- Lean dairy products
- Nuts, seeds, legumes

In small amounts:

- Alcohol
- Coffee
- Animal fats, especially red meat
- Sweets and sugar

What To Avoid

- Ready meals and canned food
- Sausages
- Bakery products
- Hydrogenated vegetable fats such as palm fat
- Sunflower oil (poor omega3 / 6 ratio)
- Pickled and smoked foods

Tips For Success

No question about it, humans need salt to survive. However, too much salt has considerable health disadvantages. In today's diet, salt is often completely overdone. This particularly applies to processed products and canned goods, junk food of all kinds, such as pizza (salami pizza 1.4 g salt per 100 g), French fries, chips, pickles and salty snacks (pretzel sticks 4.5 g salt per 100 g pretzel sticks).

But there are also plenty of hidden sources of salt, such as bread (an average of 1.3 g of salt per 100 g of bread) and rolls, meat and sausages (5.3 g of salt in 100 g of smoked ham; 3.4 g of salt in 100 g of salami), Dairy products and cheese (2.8 g salt in 40% Gouda; 2.8 g salt in 100 g feta) or in instant soups as a flavor enhancer.

Look for an alternative with less salt

If you are used to a very salty taste, you should try to switch to low-salt foods gradually. There are low-salt alternatives to many foods.

Lower salt cheeses:

- Cream cheese (1 g salt / 100 g), double cream setting
- Emmentaler 45% (0.9 g salt / 100 g)
- Mozzarella (0.5 g salt / 100 g)

Low-salt sausages:

- Cooked ham (2.5 g salt / 100 g)
- Turkey salami (3.2 g salt / 100 g)
- Mortadella (1.7 g salt / 100 g)
- Fine liver sausage (1.7 g salt / 100 g)
- Turkey breast (3.1 g salt / 100 g)
- Low-salt snacks
- Sesame sticks (0.8 g salt / 100 g)
- Cheese biscuits (0.5 g salt / 100 g)

Select another cooking method

In contrast to cooking or frying, less natural aromas are lost when steaming. This means the food retains its natural flavors and you need less salt. Choosing another cooking method will drastically reduce salt consumption. This is particularly interesting for meat, fish and vegetables.

Avoid ready meals

Ready meals take one of the foremost places in salt consumption. Even if it takes some time and effort, the best and healthiest thing to do is to cook on your own.

Salt substitute for potatoes

Especially fresh potatoes from the market and new potatoes have an excellent taste of their own. By seasoning it with rosemary, pepper and olive oil you can largely do without salt.

Salt substitute for fish

For seasoning fish dishes, dill, peppers and chilies are good (use sparingly) instead of salt. This sometimes makes the fish taste even more intense.

Salt substitute for salad

Salt can be easily replaced in the salad with your own herbal mixtures, such as basil, wild garlic, parsley, oregano, chives, watercress, garlic and oregano.

Food/Shopping List

Low GI Vegetables (1st Choice)

(3-servings/ day)

Artichokes

Aubergine

Avocados

Cauliflower

Broccoli

Green beans

Kale

Cucumbers

Cabbage

Pumpkin (summer squash)

Swiss chard

Paprika

Mushrooms

Radishes

Brussels sprouts

Arugula

Salad (the darker the green, the better)

Celery

Mustard seeds

Asparagus

Spinach

Sprouts

Zucchini

Sweet peas

Onions

Medium GI Vegetables (2nd Choice)

Peas

Potatoes (jacket potatoes)

Chickpeas

Pumpkin (butternut squash)

Pumpkin (acorn gourd)

Pumpkin (spaghetti squash)

Carrots

Sweet potatoes

Tomatoes

Low GI fruits (1st choice)

(2-servings / day)

Apples

Apricots

Bananas

Blueberries

Blackberries

Strawberries

Guava

Raspberries

Melon (honeydew melon)

Melon (cantaloupe melon)

Melon (watermelon)

Nectarines

Papayas

Peaches

Cranberries

Rhubarb

Grapes

Lemons

Medium GI fruits (2nd choice)

Pears

Figs

Grapefruit

Cherries

Kiwi fruit

Pumpkin

Tangerine

Mango

Oranges

Plums

Meat and seafood (recommended)

All fish (especially salmon, plaice, herring,

Tuna, halibut, sole, carp,

Sardines, mackerel)

All shellfish

Eggs

Chicken (skinless)

Lamb (lean)

Turkey meat (skinless)

Beef (lean and steaks)... rare!

Pork (lean and steaks)... rare!

Sausage (only lean cold cuts)

Dairy products (recommended)

Blue cheese

Butter substitute (e.g. ghee)

Buttermilk

Feta cheese

Cream cheese (low in fat)

Greek yogurt

Oat milk

Harzer cheese

Cottage Cheese and Cheddar (Low Fat)

Yogurt (low fat)

Coconut water

Almond milk

Milk (cow's milk, low-fat)

Mozzarella (low fat)

Parmesan cheese

Provolone; Italian sliced cheese (low in fat)

Rice milk

Ricotta cheese (low fat)

Sour cream (low fat)

Sliced cheese (up to 45% fat)

Swiss cheese

Soy milk

Quark (lean)

Dairy products (not recommended)

Butter

Crème fraîche and sour cream

Fruit curd

Mayonnaise

Milk (full fat)

Rice pudding

Pudding

Cream

Fats / oils (approx. 2 tbsp. / day)

Coconut oil

Flaxseed oil

Olive oil

Rapeseed oil

Nuts, seeds, etc. (approx. 20 g / day)

Cashew nuts

Hazelnuts

Pumpkin seeds

Macadamia

Almonds

Pine nuts

Sesame seeds

Sunflower seeds

Walnuts

Nuts, seeds (not recommended)

Peanuts

All salted nuts

Cereal products (recommended)

Amaranth

Dark Bread

Barley

Oatmeal

Cornbread

Almond flour

Muesli without sugar

Pasta (whole grain)

Quinoa

Rice (whole grain)

Whole wheat pita

Whole grain tortillas

Whole grain bread

Wholegrain crisp bread

Whole wheat flour

Wheat germ

Cereal products (not recommended)

Croissants

Durum wheat pasta

Potato pancakes

Croquettes

Pancakes

French fries

Rice (peeled)

White bread

Wheat and milk rolls

Zwieback

Snacks (recommended)

Olives

Dried fruits (without sugar)

Dates

Vegetable sticks

Snacks (not recommended)

Sweet and salty baked goods

Sweets

Savory biscuits (chips, flips etc.)

Sweet dairy products (fruit yogurt, etc.)

Drinks (recommended) - 2-3 l / day

Fruit juice (freshly squeezed)

Green tea

herbal tea

Water

Drinks (not recommended)

Alcohol

Fruit juices (ready-made juices)

Coffee

Black tea

Soft drinks

CHAPTER 3:

Breakfast

Sweet Potatoes With Coconut Flakes

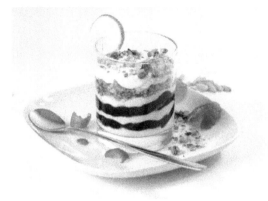

Preparation time: 15 minutes

Cooking time: 1 hour

Servings: 2

Ingredients:

- 16 oz. sweet potatoes

- 1 tbsp. maple syrup

- 1/4 c. Fat-free coconut Greek yogurt

- 1/8 c. unsweetened toasted coconut flakes

- 1 chopped apple

Directions:

1. Preheat oven to 400 0F.

2. Place your potatoes on a baking sheet. Bake them for 45 - 60 minutes or until soft.

3. Use a sharp knife to mark "X" on the potatoes and fluff pulp with a fork.

4. Top with coconut flakes, chopped apple, Greek yogurt, and maple syrup.

5. Serve immediately.

Nutrition:

Calories: 321, Fat: 3 g Carbs: 70 g

Protein: 7 g Sugars: 0.1 g Sodium: 3%

Flaxseed & Banana Smoothie

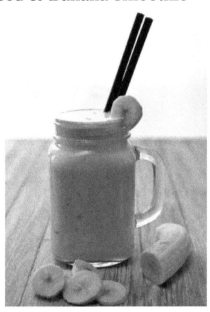

Preparation time: 5 minutes

Cooking time: 0 minutes

Servings: 1

Ingredients:

- 1 frozen banana

- 1/2 c. almond milk

- Vanilla extract.

- 1 tbsp. almond butter

- 2 tbsps. Flaxseed

- 1 tsp. maple syrup

Directions:

1. Add all your ingredients to a food processor or blender and run until smooth. Pour the mixture into a glass and enjoy.

Nutrition:

Calories: 376, Fat: 19.4 g Carbs: 48.3 g

Protein: 9.2 g Sugars: 12% Sodium: 64.9 mg

Fruity Tofu Smoothie

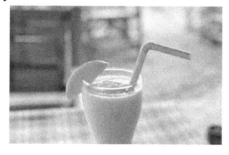

Preparation time: 5 minutes

Cooking time: 0 minutes

Servings: 2

Ingredients:

- 1 c. ice cold water

- 1 c. packed spinach

- 1/4 c. frozen mango chunks

- 1/2 c. frozen pineapple chunks

- 1 tbsp. chia seeds

- 1 container silken tofu

- 1 frozen medium banana

Directions:

1. In a powerful blender, add all ingredients and puree until smooth and creamy.

2. Evenly divide into two glasses, serve and enjoy.

Nutrition: Calories: 175, Fat: 3.7 g

Carbs: 33.3 g Protein: 6.0 g

Sugars: 16.3 g Sodium: 1%

French Toast With Applesauce

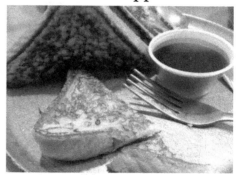

Preparation time: 5 minutes

Cooking time: 5 minutes

Servings: 6

Ingredients:

- 1/4 c. unsweetened applesauce

- 1/2 c. skim milk

- 2 packets Stevia

- 2 eggs

- 6 slices whole wheat bread

- 1 tsp. ground cinnamon

Directions:

1. Mix well applesauce, sugar, cinnamon, milk and eggs in a mixing bowl.

2. One slice at a time, soak the bread into applesauce mixture until wet.

3. On medium fire, heat a large nonstick skillet.

4. Add soaked bread on one side and another on the other side. Cook in a single layer in batches for 2-3 minutes per side on medium low fire or until lightly browned.

5. Serve and enjoy.

Nutrition:

Calories: 122.6, Fat: 2.6 g

Carbs: 18.3 g Protein: 6.5 g

Sugars: 14.8 g Sodium: 11%

Banana-Peanut Butter 'N Greens Smoothie

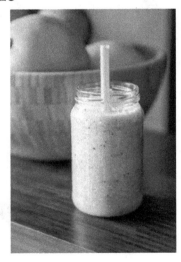

Preparation time: 5 minutes

Cooking time: 0 minutes

Servings: 1

Ingredients:

- 1 c. chopped and packed Romaine lettuce

- 1 frozen medium banana

- 1 tbsp. all-natural peanut butter

- 1 c. cold almond milk

Directions:

1. In a heavy-duty blender, add all ingredients.

2. Puree until smooth and creamy.

3. Serve and enjoy.

Nutrition:

Calories: 349.3, Fat: 9.7 g

Carbs: 57.4 g Protein: 8.1 g

Sugars: 4.3 g Sodium: 18%

Baking Powder Biscuits

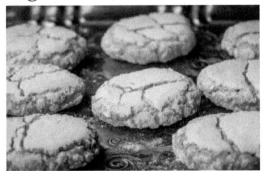

Preparation time: 5 minutes

Cooking time: 5 minutes

Servings: 1

Ingredients:

- 1 egg white

- 1 c. white whole-wheat flour

- 4 tbsps. Non-hydrogenated vegetable shortening

- 1 tbsp. sugar

- 2/3 c. low-

- Fat free milk

- 1 c. unbleached all-purpose flour

- 4 tsps. Sodium-free baking powder

Directions:

1. Preheat oven to 450°F. Take out a baking sheet and set aside.

2. Place the flour, sugar, and baking powder into a mixing bowl and whisk well to combine.

3. Cut the shortening into the mixture using your fingers, and work until it resembles coarse crumbs. Add the egg white and milk and stir to combine.

4. Turn the dough out onto a lightly floured surface and knead 1 minute. Roll dough to ¾ inch thickness and cut into 12 rounds.

5. Place rounds on the baking sheet. Place baking sheet on middle rack in oven and bake 10 minutes.

6. Remove baking sheet and place biscuits on a wire rack to cool.

Nutrition: Calories: 118, Fat: 4 g Carbs: 16 g

Protein: 3 g Sugars: 0.2 g Sodium: 6%

Oatmeal Banana Pancakes With Walnuts

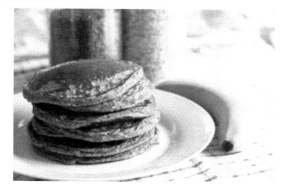

Preparation time: 15 minutes

Cooking time: 5 minutes

Servings: 8 pancakes

Ingredients:

- 1 finely diced firm banana

- 1 c. whole wheat pancake mix

- 1/8 c. chopped walnuts

- 1/4 c. old-fashioned oats

Directions:

1. Make the pancake mix according to the directions on the package.

2. Add walnuts, oats, and chopped banana.

3. Coat a griddle with cooking spray. Add about 1/4 cup of the pancake batter onto the griddle when hot.

4. Turn pancake over when bubbles form on top. Cook until golden brown.

5. Serve immediately.

Nutrition:

Calories: 155 Fat: 4 g Carbs: 28 g

Protein: 7 g Sugars: 2.2 g Sodium: 10%

Creamy Oats, Greens & Blueberry Smoothie

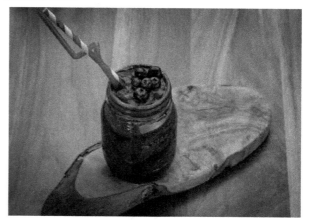

Preparation time: 4 minutes

Cooking time: 0 minutes

Servings: 1

Ingredients:

- 1 c. cold

- Fat-free milk

- 1 c. salad greens

- 1/2 c. fresh frozen blueberries

- 1/2 c. frozen cooked oatmeal

- 1 tbsp. sunflower seeds

Directions:

1. In a powerful blender, blend all ingredients until smooth and creamy.

2. Serve and enjoy.

Nutrition: Calories: 280,

Fat: 6.8 g Carbs: 44.0 g

Protein: 14.0 g Sugars: 32 g

Sodium: 141%

Banana & Cinnamon Oatmeal

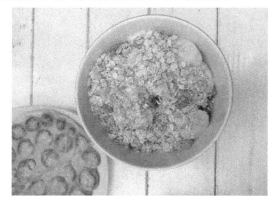

Preparation time: 5 minutes

Cooking time: 0 minutes

Servings: 6

Ingredients:

- 2 c. quick-cooking oats

- 4 c. Fat-free milk

- 1 tsp. ground cinnamon

- 2 chopped large ripe banana

- 4 tsps. Brown sugar

- Extra ground cinnamon

Directions:

1. Place milk in a skillet and bring to boil. Add oats and cook over medium heat until thickened, for two to four minutes. Stir intermittently.

2. Add cinnamon, brown sugar and banana and stir to combine.

3. If you want, serve with the extra cinnamon and milk. Enjoy!

Nutrition: Calories: 215, Fat: 2 g Carbs: 42 g

Protein: 10 g Sugars: 1 g Sodium: 40%

Bagels Made Healthy

Preparation time: 5 minutes

Cooking time: 40 minutes

Servings: 8

Ingredients:

- 1 1/2 c. warm water

- 1 1/4 c. bread flour

- 2 tbsps. Honey

- 2 c. whole wheat flour

- 2 tsps. Yeast

- 1 1/2 tbsps. Olive oil

- 1 tbsp. vinegar

Directions:

1. In a bread machine, mix all ingredients, and then process on dough cycle.

2. Once done, create 8 pieces shaped like a flattened ball.

3. Make a hole in the center of each ball using your thumb then create a donut shape.

4. In a greased baking sheet, place donut-shaped dough then cover and let it rise about 1/2 hour.

5. Prepare about 2 inches of water to boil in a large pan.

6. In boiling water, drop one at a time the bagels and boil for 1 minute, then turn them once.

7. Remove them and return to baking sheet and bake at 350F for about 20 to 25 minutes until golden brown.

Nutrition:

Calories: 228.1, Fat: 3.7 g Carbs: 41.8 g

Protein: 6.9 g Sugars: 0 g Sodium: 15%

Cereal With Cranberry-Orange Twist

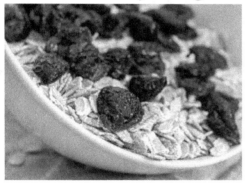

Preparation time: 5 minutes

Cooking time: 0 minutes

Servings: 1

Ingredients:

- 1/2 c. water

- 1/2 c. orange juice

- 1/3 c. oat bran

- 1/4 c. dried cranberries

- Sugar

- Milk

Directions:

1. In a bowl, combine all ingredients.

2. For about 2 minutes, microwave the bowl then serve with sugar and milk.

3. Enjoy!

Nutrition:

Calories: 220.4, Fat: 2.4 g Carbs: 43.5 g

Protein: 6.2 g Sugars: 8 g Sodium: 1%

No Cook Overnight Oats

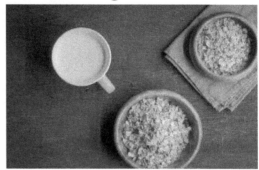

Preparation time: 5 minutes

Cooking time: 0 minutes

Servings: 1

Ingredients:

- 1 1/2 c. low Fat milk

- 5 whole almond pieces

- 1 tsp. chia seeds

- 2 tbsps. Oats

- 1 tsp. sunflower seeds

- 1 tbsp. Raisins

Directions:

1. In a jar or mason bottle with cap, mix all ingredients.

2. Refrigerate overnight.

3. Enjoy for breakfast. Will keep in the fridge for up to 3 days.

Nutrition: Calories: 271, Fat: 9.8 g Carbs: 35.4 g Protein: 16.7 g Sodium: 103%

Avocado Cup With Egg

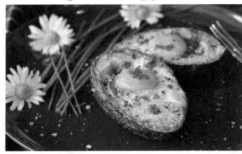

Preparation time: 5 minutes

Cooking time: 0 minutes

Servings: 4

Ingredients:

- 4 tsps. Parmesan cheese

- 1 chopped stalk scallion

- 4 dashes pepper

- 4 dashes paprika

- 2 ripe avocados

- 4 medium eggs

Directions:

1. Preheat oven to 375F.

2. Slice avocadoes in half and discard seed.

3. Slice the rounded portions of the avocado, to make it level and sit well on a baking sheet.

4. Place avocadoes on baking sheet and crack one egg in each hole of the avocado.

5. Season each egg evenly with pepper, and paprika.

6. Pop in the oven and bake for 25 minutes or until eggs are cooked to your liking.

7. Serve with a sprinkle of Parmesan.

Nutrition:

Calories: 206,

Fat: 15.4 g Carbs: 11.3 g

Protein: 8.5 g Sugars: 0.4 g

Sodium: 21%

Mediterranean Toast

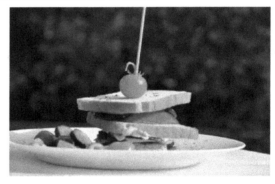

Preparation time: 10 minutes

Servings: 2

Cooking time: 0 minutes

Ingredients:

- 1 1/2 tsp. reduced-Fat crumbled feta

- 3 sliced Greek olives

- 1/4 mashed avocado

- 1 slice good whole wheat bread

- 1 tbsp. roasted red pepper hummus

- 3 sliced cherry tomatoes

- 1 sliced hardboiled egg

Directions:

1. First, toast the bread and top it with 1/4 mashed avocado and 1 tablespoon hummus.

2. Add the cherry tomatoes, olives, hardboiled egg and feta.

3. To taste, season with salt and pepper.

Nutrition:

Calories: 333.7

Fat: 17 g

Carbs: 33.3 g

Protein: 16.3 g

Sugars: 1 g

Sodium: 19%

Instant Banana Oatmeal

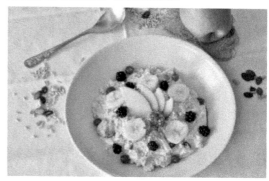

Preparation time: 1 min

Servings: 1

Cooking time: 0 minutes

Ingredients:

- 1 mashed ripe banana

- 1/2 c. water

- 1/2 c. quick oats

Directions:

1. Measure the oats and water into a microwave-safe bowl and stir to combine.

2. Place bowl in microwave and heat on high for 2 minutes.

3. Remove bowl from microwave and stir in the mashed banana and enjoy.

Nutrition:

Calories: 243

Fat: 3 g

Carbs: 50 g

Protein: 6 g

Sugars: 20 g

Sodium: 30 mg

CHAPTER 4:

Lunch

Corn And Beans Tortillas

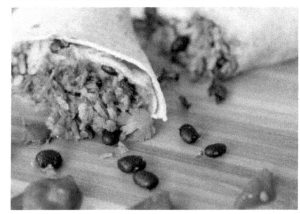

Preparation time: 5 minutes

Cooking time: 12 minutes

Servings: 4

Ingredients:

- 1 cup canned black beans, no-salt-added, drained and rinsed
- 1 green bell pepper, chopped
- 1 carrots, peeled and grated
- 1 tablespoon olive oil
- 1 red onion, sliced
- 1/2 cup corn
- 1 cup low-fat cheddar, shredded
- 6 whole wheat tortillas
- 1 cup non-fat yogurt

Directions:

1. Heat up a pan with the oil over medium heat; and sauté the onion for 2 minutes.
2. Add the beans, carrot, bell pepper and the corn, stir, and cook for 10 minutes more.

3. Arrange the tortillas on a working surface, divide the beans mix on each, also divide the cheese and the yogurt, roll and serve for lunch.

Nutrition: 478 calories, 24.9g protein, 78.4g carbohydrates, 9.1g fat, 13.8g fiber, 11mg cholesterol, 375mg sodium, 1072mg potassium

Chicken And Spinach Mix

Preparation time: 10 minutes

Cooking time: 20 minutes

Servings: 4

Ingredients:

- 2 chicken breasts, skinless, boneless and cubed
- 1/4 cup low-sodium chicken stock
- 1/2 cup celery, chopped
- 1 cup baby spinach
- 1 mango, peeled, and cubed
- 2 spring onions, chopped
- 1 tablespoon olive oil
- 1 teaspoon thyme, dried
- 1/4 teaspoon garlic powder
- A pinch of black pepper

Directions:

1. Heat up a pan with the oil over medium-high heat, add the spring onions and the chicken and brown for 5 minutes.
2. Add the celery and the other ingredients except the spinach, toss and cook for 12 minutes more.

3. Add the spinach, toss, cook for 2-3 minutes, divide everything between plates and serve.

Nutrition: 227 calories, 22.4g protein, 14.1g carbohydrates, 9.3g fat, 2g fiber, 65mg cholesterol, 89mg sodium, 418mg potassium

Garlic Chickpeas Fritters

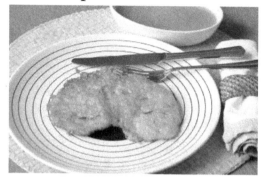

Preparation time: 10 minutes

Cooking time: 10 minutes

Servings: 4

Ingredients:

- 2 garlic cloves, minced
- 15 ounces canned chickpeas, no-salt-added, drained and rinsed
- 1 teaspoon chili powder
- 1 teaspoon cumin, ground
- 1 egg
- 1 tablespoon olive oil
- 1 tablespoon lime juice
- 1 tablespoon lime zest, grated
- 1 tablespoon cilantro, chopped

Directions:

1. In a blender, combine the chickpeas with the garlic and the other ingredients except the egg and pulse well.
2. Shape medium cakes out of this mix.
3. Heat up a pan with the oil over medium-high heat, add the chickpeas cakes, cook for 5 minutes on each

side, divide between plates and serve for lunch with a side salad.

Nutrition: 440 calories, 22.2g protein, 65.9g carbohydrates, 11.3g fat, 19g fiber, 41mg cholesterol, 49mg sodium, 977mg potassium

Cheddar Cauliflower Bowls

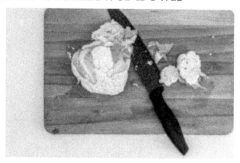

Preparation time: 10 minutes

Cooking time: 10 minutes

Servings: 4

Ingredients:

- 1 tablespoon avocado oil
- 1 cup red bell peppers, cubed
- 1 pound cauliflower florets
- 1 red onion, chopped
- 3 tablespoons salsa
- 2 tablespoons low-fat cheddar, shredded
- 2 tablespoons coconut cream

Directions:

1. Heat up a pan with the oil over medium-high heat; add the onion and peppers, and sauté for 2 minutes.
2. Add the cauliflower and the other ingredients, and then toss, cook for 8 minutes more, divide into bowls and serve.

Nutrition: 79 calories, 4.4g protein, 12.5g carbohydrates, 2.5g fat, 4.3g fiber, 1mg cholesterol, 134mg sodium, 506mg potassium

Salmon Salad

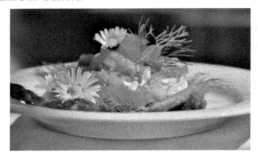

Preparation time: 5 minutes

Cooking time: 0 minutes

Servings: 4

Ingredients:

- 1 cup canned salmon, drained and flaked
- 1 tablespoon lime zest, grated
- 1 tablespoon lime juice
- 3 tablespoons fat-free yogurt
- 1 cup baby spinach
- 1 teaspoon capers, drained and chopped
- 1 red onion, chopped
- A pinch of black pepper
- 1 tablespoon chives, chopped

Directions:

1. In a bowl, combine the salmon with lime zest, lime juice and the other ingredients, toss and serve cold for lunch.

Nutrition: 67 calories, 9.2g protein, 4.1g carbohydrates, 1.5g fat, 1g fiber, 21mg cholesterol, 64mg sodium, 245mg potassium

Chicken And Tomato Mix

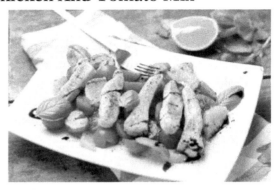

Preparation time: 10 minutes

Cooking time: 20 minutes

Servings: 4

Ingredients:

- 1 tablespoon olive oil
- 1 pound chicken breast, skinless, boneless and cubed
- 1/2 pound kale, torn
- 2 cherry tomatoes, halved
- 1 yellow onion, chopped
- 1/2 cup low-sodium chicken stock
- 1/4 cup low-fat mozzarella, shredded

Directions:

1. Heat up a pan with the oil over medium heat, add the chicken and the onion and brown for 5 minutes.
2. Add the kale and the other ingredients accept the mozzarella, toss, and cook for 12 minute more.
3. Sprinkle the cheese on top, cook the mix for 2-3 minutes, divide between plates and serve for lunch.

Nutrition: 230 calories, 28.2g protein, 11.1g carbohydrates, 7.7g fat, 2.2g fiber, 78mg cholesterol, 158mg sodium, 884mg potassium

Salmon And Olives Salad

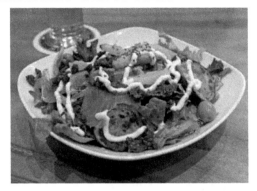

Preparation time: 10 minutes

Cooking time: 0 minutes

Servings: 4

Ingredients:

- 6 ounces canned salmon, drained and cubed
- 1 tablespoon balsamic vinegar
- 1 tablespoon olive oil
- 2 shallots, chopped
- 1/2 cup black olives, pitted and halved
- 2 cups baby arugula
- A pinch of black pepper

Directions:

1. In a bowl, combine the salmon with the shallots and the other ingredients, toss and keep in the fridge for 10 minutes before serving for lunch.

Nutrition: 116 calories, 8.9g protein, 3.1g carbohydrates, 8g fat, 0.7g fiber, 19mg cholesterol, 169mg sodium, 238mg potassium

Shrimp Salad

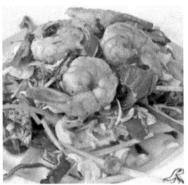

Preparation time: 5 minutes

Cooking time: 10 minutes

Servings: 4

Ingredients:

- 1 tablespoon olive oil
- 1 pound shrimp, peeled and deveined
- 1 tablespoon basil pesto
- 1 cup baby arugula
- 1 yellow onion, chopped
- 1 cucumber, sliced
- 1 cup carrots, shredded
- 1 tablespoon cilantro, chopped

Directions:

1. Heat up a pan with the oil over medium heat, then add the onion and carrots, stir and cook for 3 minutes.
2. Add the shrimp and the other ingredients, toss, cook for 7 minutes more, divide into bowls and serve.

Nutrition: 200 calories, 27g protein, 9.9g carbohydrates, 5.6g fat, 1.8g fiber, 239mg cholesterol, 300mg sodium, 452mg potassium

Turkey Tortillas

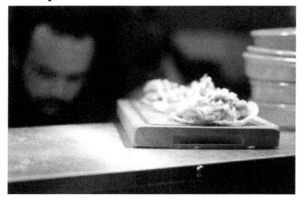

Preparation time: 10 minutes

Cooking time: 3 minutes

Servings: 2

Ingredients:

- 2 whole wheat tortillas
- 2 teaspoons mustard
- 2 teaspoons mayonnaise
- 1 turkey breast, skinless, boneless and cut into strips
- 1 tablespoons olive oil
- 1 red onion, chopped
- 1 red bell peppers, cut into strips
- 1 green bell pepper, cut into strips
- 1/4 cup low-fat mozzarella, shredded

Directions:

1. Heat up a pan with the oil over medium heat, add the meat and the onion and brown for 5 minutes
2. Add the peppers, toss and cook for 10 minutes more.
3. Arrange the tortillas on a working surface, divide the turkey mix on each, also divide the mayo, mustard and the cheese, wrap and serve for lunch.

Nutrition: 303 calories, 15.9g protein, 37.8g carbohydrates, 11.1g fat, 7g fiber, 15mg cholesterol, 620mg sodium, 394mg potassium

Parsley Green Beans Soup

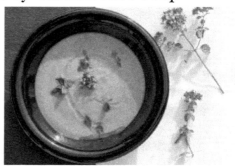

Preparation time: 5 minutes

Cooking time: 25 minutes

Servings: 4

Ingredients:

- 2 teaspoons olive oil
- 2 garlic cloves, minced
- 1 pound green beans, trimmed and halved
- 1 yellow onion, chopped
- 2 tomatoes, cubed
- 1 teaspoon sweet paprika
- 1 quart low-sodium chicken stock
- 2 tablespoons parsley, chopped

Directions:

1. Heat up a pot with the oil over medium-high heat; add the garlic and the onion, stir and sauté for 5 minutes.
2. Add the green beans and the other ingredients except the parsley, stir, bring to a simmer and cook for 20 minutes.
3. Add the parsley, stir, divide the soup into bowls and serve.

Nutrition: 87 calories, 4.1g protein, 14g carbohydrates, 2.7g fat, 5.5g fiber, 0mg cholesterol, 147mg sodium, 452mg potassium

Beef Skillet

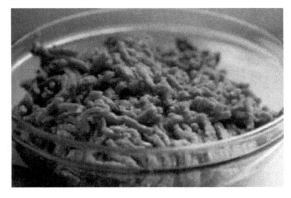

Preparation time: 5 minutes

Cooking time: 20 minutes

Servings: 4

Ingredients:

- 1 pound beef, ground
- 1/2 cup yellow onion, chopped
- 1 tablespoon olive oil
- 1 cup zucchini, cubed
- 2 garlic cloves, minced
- 14 ounces canned tomatoes, no-salt-added, chopped
- 1 teaspoon Italian seasoning
- 1/4 cup low-fat parmesan, shredded
- 1 tablespoon chives, chopped
- 1 tablespoon cilantro, chopped

Directions:

1. Heat up a pan with the oil over medium heat, add the garlic, onion and the beef and brown for 5 minutes.
2. Add the rest of the ingredients, toss, cook for 15 minutes more, divide into bowls and serve for lunch.

Nutrition: 300 calories, 37.2g protein, 9.3g carbohydrates, 12.5g fat, 1.9g fiber, 108mg cholesterol, 184mg sodium, 797mg potassium

Thyme Beef And Tomatoes

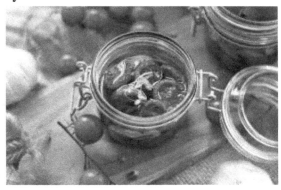

Preparation time: 10 minutes

Cooking time: 25 minutes

Servings: 4

Ingredients:

- 1/2 pound beef, ground
- 3 tablespoons olive oil
- 1 and ¾ pounds red potatoes, peeled and roughly cubed
- 1 yellow onion, chopped
- 2 teaspoons thyme, dried
- 1 cup canned tomatoes, no-salt-added, and chopped
- A pinch of black pepper

Directions:

1. Heat up a pan with the oil over medium-high heat
2. Add the onion and the beef, stir and brown for 5 minutes.
3. Add the potatoes and the rest of the ingredients, toss, bring to a simmer, cook for 20 minutes more, divide into bowls and serve for lunch.

Nutrition: 355 calories, 21.7g protein, 36.2g carbohydrates, 14.5g fat, 4.7g fiber, 51mg cholesterol, 53mg sodium, 1282mg potassium

Pork Soup

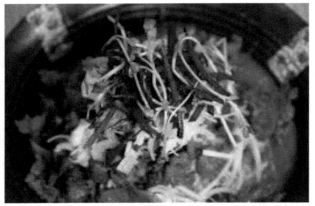

Preparation time: 10 minutes

Cooking time: 25 minutes

Servings: 4

Ingredients:

- 1 tablespoon olive oil
- 1 red onion, chopped
- 1 pound pork stew meat, cubed
- 1 quart low-sodium beef stock
- 1 pound carrots, sliced
- 1 cup tomato puree
- 1 tablespoon cilantro, chopped

Directions:

1. Heat up a pot with the oil in medium-high heat, add the onion and the meat and brown for five minutes.
2. Add the rest of the ingredients except the cilantro, bring to a simmer, reduce heat to medium, and boil the soup for 20 minutes.
3. Ladle into bowls and serve for lunch with the cilantro sprinkled on top.

Nutrition: 354 calories, 36g protein, 19.3g carbohydrates, 14.6g fat, 4.6g fiber, 98mg cholesterol, 199mg sodium, 1104mg potassium

Shrimp And Spinach Salad

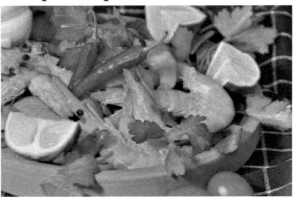

Preparation time: 5 minutes

Cooking time: 7 minutes

Servings: 4

Ingredients:

- 1 cup corn
- 1 endive, shredded
- 1 cup baby spinach
- 1 pound shrimp, peeled and deveined
- 2 garlic cloves, minced
- 1 tablespoon lime juice
- 2 cups strawberries, halved
- 2 tablespoons olive oil
- 2 tablespoons balsamic vinegar
- 1 tablespoon cilantro, chopped

Directions:

1. Heat up a pan with the oil over medium-high heat, add the garlic and brown for 1 minute. Add the shrimp and lime juice, toss and cook for 3 minutes on each side.
2. In a salad bowl, combine the shrimp with the corn, endive and the other ingredients, toss and serve for lunch.

Nutrition: 257 calories, 28g protein, 15.6g carbohydrates, 9.6g fat, 2.9g fiber, 239mg cholesterol, 291mg sodium, 481mg potassium

Raspberry Shrimp And Tomato Salad

Preparation time: 5 minutes

Cooking time: 10 minutes

Servings: 4

Ingredients:

- 1 pound green beans, trimmed and halved
- 2 tablespoons olive oil
- 2 pounds shrimp, peeled and deveined
- 1 tablespoon lemon juice
- 2 cups cherry tomatoes, halved
- 1/4 cup raspberry vinegar
- A pinch of black pepper

Directions:

1. Heat up a pan with the oil over medium-high heat, add the shrimp, toss and cook for 2 minutes.
2. Add the green beans and the other ingredients, toss, cook for 8 minutes more, divide into bowls and serve for lunch.

Nutrition: 379 calories, 53.9g protein, 13g carbohydrates, 11.1g fat, 4g fiber, 478mg cholesterol, 574mg sodium, 613mg potassium

CHAPTER 5:

Dinner

Cod Tacos

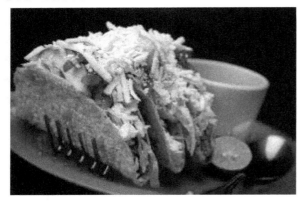

Preparation time: 10 minutes

Cooking time: 10 minutes

Servings: 2

Ingredients:

- 4 whole wheat taco shells
- 1 tablespoon light mayonnaise
- 1 tablespoon salsa
- 1 tablespoon low-fat mozzarella, shredded
- 1 tablespoon olive oil
- 1 red onion, chopped
- 1 tablespoon cilantro, chopped
- 2 cod fillets, boneless, skinless and cubed
- 1 tablespoon tomato puree

Directions:

1. Heat up a pan with oil over medium heat, add the onions, stir and cook for 2 minutes.
2. Add the fish and tomato puree, toss gently and cook for 5 minutes more.

3. Spoon this into the taco shells, also divide the mayo, salsa and the cheese and serve for lunch.

Nutrition: 454 calories, 31.7g protein, 56.1g carbohydrates, 14.5g fat, 7.5g fiber, 38mg cholesterol, 487mg sodium, 142mg potassium

Zucchini Fritters

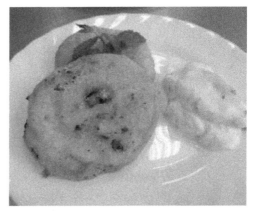

Preparation time: 10 minutes

Cooking time: 10 minutes

Servings: 4

Ingredients:

- 1 yellow onion, chopped
- 2 zucchinis, grated
- 2 tablespoons almond flour
- 1 egg, whisked
- 1 garlic clove, minced
- A pinch of black pepper
- 1/3 cup carrot, shredded
- 1/3 cup low-fat cheddar, grated
- 1 tablespoon cilantro, chopped

- 1 teaspoon lemon zest, grated
- 2 tablespoons olive oil

Directions:

1. In a bowl, combine the zucchinis with the garlic, onion and the other ingredients except the oil, stir well and shape medium cakes out of this mix.
2. Heat up a pan with the oil over medium-high heat, add the zucchini cakes, cook for 5 minutes on each side, divide between plates and serve with a side salad.

Nutrition: 204 calories, 8.3g protein, 10.4g carbohydrates, 16g fat, 3.5g fiber, 43mg cholesterol, 96mg sodium, 353mg potassium

Chickpeas Stew

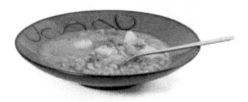

Preparation time: 10 minutes

Cooking time: 20 minutes

Servings: 4

Ingredients:

- 1 tablespoon olive oil
- 1 yellow onion, chopped
- 2 teaspoons chili powder
- 14 ounces canned chickpeas, no-salt-added, drained and rinsed
- 14 ounces canned tomatoes, no-salt-added, cubed
- 1 cup low-sodium chicken stock
- 1 tablespoon cilantro, chopped

- A pinch of black pepper

Directions:

1. Heat up a pot with the oil over medium-high heat, add the onion and chili powder, stir and cook for 5 minutes.
2. Add the chickpeas and the other ingredients, toss, cook for 15 minutes over medium heat, divide into bowls and serve for lunch.

Nutrition: 425 calories, 20.7g protein, 67.3g carbohydrates, 9.9g fat, 19.5g fiber, 0mg cholesterol, 77mg sodium, 1170mg potassium

Lemon Chicken Salad

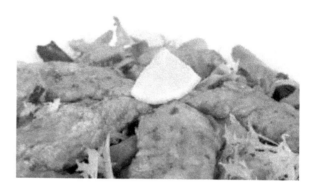

Preparation time: 10 minutes

Cooking time: 0 minutes

Servings: 4

Ingredients:

- 1 tablespoon olive oil
- A pinch of black pepper
- 2 rotisserie chicken, skinless, boneless, shredded
- 1 pound cherry tomatoes, halved
- 1 red onion, chopped
- 4 cups baby spinach
- 1/4 cup walnuts, chopped
- 1/2 teaspoon lemon zest, grated
- 2 tablespoons lemon juice

Directions:

1. In a salad bowl, combine the chicken with the tomato and the other ingredients, toss and serve for lunch.

Nutrition: 199 calories, 21.6g protein, 10.6g carbohydrates, 9.1g fat, 3.2g fiber, 53mg cholesterol, 292mg sodium, 527mg potassium

Asparagus Salad

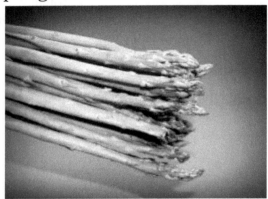

Preparation time: 10 minutes

Cooking time: 20 minutes

Servings: 4

Ingredients:

- 3 garlic cloves, minced
- 2 tablespoons olive oil
- 1 red onion, chopped
- 3 carrots, sliced
- 1/2 cup low-sodium chicken stock
- 2 cups baby spinach
- 1 pound asparagus, trimmed and halved
- 1 red bell pepper, cut into strips
- 1 yellow bell pepper, cut into strips
- 1 green bell pepper, cut into strips
- A pinch of black pepper

Directions:

1. Heat up a pan with the oil over medium heat

2. Add the onion and the garlic, stir it and sauté for two minutes.
3. Add the asparagus and the other ingredients except the spinach, toss, and cook for 15 minutes.
4. Add the spinach, cook everything for 3 minutes more, divide into bowls and serve for lunch.

Nutrition: 141 calories, 4.7g protein, 17.8g carbohydrates, 7.4g fat, 5.9g fiber, 0mg cholesterol, 66mg sodium, 669mg potassium

Tomato Beef Stew

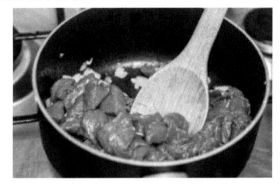

Preparation time: 10 minutes

Cooking time: 1 hour and 20 minutes

Servings: 4

Ingredients:

- 1 pound beef stew meat, cubed
- 1 cup no-salt-added tomato sauce
- 1 cup low-sodium beef stock
- 1 tablespoon olive oil
- 1 yellow onion, chopped
- 1/4 teaspoon hot sauce
- 1 teaspoon onion powder
- 1 teaspoon garlic powder
- 1 tablespoon cilantro, chopped

Directions:

1. Heat up a pot with the oil over medium-high heat, add the meat and the onion, stir and brown for 5 minutes.

2. Add the tomato sauce and the rest of the ingredients bring to a simmer and cook over medium heat for 1 hour and 15 minutes.
3. Divide into bowls and serve for lunch.

Nutrition: 273 calories, 36.2g protein, 6.9g carbohydrates, 10.7g fat, 1.6g fiber, 101mg cholesterol, 440mg sodium, 715mg potassium

Rosemary Pork Chops

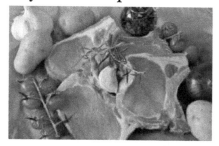

Preparation time: 5 minutes

Cooking time: 8 hours and 10 minutes

Servings: 4

Ingredients:

- 4 pork chops
- 1 tablespoon olive oil
- 2 shallots, chopped
- 1 pound white mushrooms, sliced
- 1/2 cup low-sodium beef stock
- 1 tablespoon rosemary, chopped
- 1/4 teaspoon garlic powder
- 1 teaspoon sweet paprika

Directions:

1. Heat up a pan with the oil over medium-high heat, add then the pork chops and the shallots, toss brown for 10 minutes and transfer to a slow cooker.
2. Add the rest of the ingredients, put the lid on and cook on Low for 8 hours.

3. Divide the pork chops and mushrooms between plates and serve for lunch.

Nutrition: 324 calories, 22.2g protein, 6.4g carbohydrates, 23.9g fat, 1.7g fiber, 69mg cholesterol, 82mg sodium, 692mg potassium

Balsamic Shrimp Salad

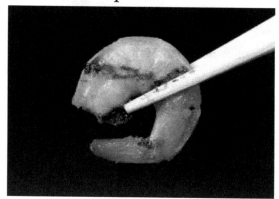

Preparation time: 10 minutes

Cooking time: 8 minutes

Servings: 4

Ingredients:

- 1 tablespoon olive oil
- 1 red onion, sliced
- 1 pound shrimp, peeled and deveined
- 2 cups baby arugula
- 1 tablespoon balsamic vinegar
- 1 tablespoon lemon juice
- 1 tablespoon coriander, chopped
- A pinch of black pepper

Directions:

1. Heat up a pan with the oil over medium heat; add then the onion, stir and sauté for 2 minutes.
2. Add the shrimp and the other ingredients, toss, cook for 6 minutes, divide into bowls and serve for lunch.

Nutrition: 180 calories, 26.4g protein, 4.8g carbohydrates, 5.6g fat, 0.8g fiber, 239mg cholesterol, 282mg sodium, 278mg potassium

Eggplant And Tomato Stew

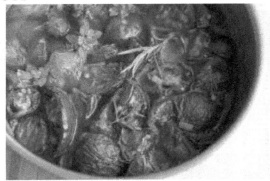

Preparation time: 5 minutes

Cooking time: 20 minutes

Servings: 4

Ingredients:

- 1 pound eggplants, roughly cubed
- 2 garlic cloves, minced
- 2 tablespoons olive oil
- 1 yellow onion, chopped
- 1 teaspoon sweet paprika
- 1/2 cup cilantro, chopped
- 14 ounces low-sodium canned tomatoes, chopped
- 1 tablespoon cilantro, chopped

Directions:

1. Heat up a pan with the oil over medium-high heat
2. Add the onion and the garlic and sauté for 2 minutes.
3. Add the eggplant and the other ingredients except the cilantro bring to a simmer and cook for 18 minutes.
4. Divide into bowls and serve with the cilantro sprinkled on top.

Nutrition: 153 calories, 2.9g protein, 18.4g carbohydrates, 8.6g fat, 6.2g fiber, 3mg cholesterol, 35mg sodium, 329mg potassium

Lime Turkey Stew

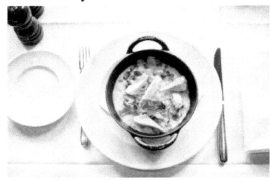

Preparation time: 5 minutes

Cooking time: 30 minutes

Servings: 4

Ingredients:

- 2 tablespoons olive oil
- 1 turkey breast, skinless, boneless and cubed
- 1 cup low-sodium beef stock
- 1 cup tomato puree
- 1/4 teaspoon lime zest, grated
- 1 yellow onion, chopped
- 1 tablespoon sweet paprika
- 1 tablespoon cilantro, chopped
- 2 tablespoons lime juice
- 1/4 teaspoon ginger, grated

Directions:

1. Heat up a pot with the oil over medium-high heat
2. Add the onion and the meat and brown for 5 minutes.
3. Add the stock and the other ingredients bring to a simmer and cook over medium heat for 25 minutes.
4. Divide the mix into bowls and serve for lunch.

Nutrition: 147 calories, 9.5g protein, 11.1g carbohydrates, 8.1g fat, 2.7g fiber, 18mg cholesterol, 491mg sodium, 488mg potassium

Beef And Beans Salad

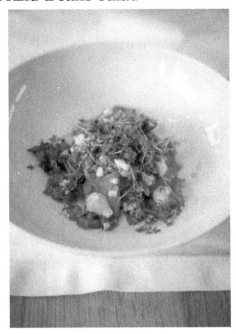

Preparation time: 10 minutes

Cooking time: 30 minutes

Servings: 4

Ingredients:

- 1 pound beef stew meat, cut into strips
- 1 tablespoon sage, chopped
- 1 tablespoon olive oil
- A pinch of black pepper
- 1/2 teaspoon cumin, ground
- 2 cups cherry tomatoes, cubed
- 1 avocado, peeled, pitted and cubed
- 1 cup canned black beans, no-salt-added, drained and rinsed
- 1/2 cup green onions, chopped
- 2 tablespoons lime juice
- 2 tablespoons balsamic vinegar
- 2 tablespoons cilantro, chopped

Directions:

1. Heat up a pan with the oil over medium-high heat, add the meat and brown for five minutes.
2. Add the sage, black pepper and the cumin, toss and cook for 5 minutes more.
3. Add the rest of the ingredients, toss, reduce heat to medium and cook the mix for 20 minutes.
4. Divide the salad into bowls and serve for lunch.

Nutrition: 533 calories, 47g protein, 39.5g carbohydrates, 21.4g fat, 12.4g fiber, 101mg cholesterol, 88mg sodium, 1686mg potassium

Squash And Peppers Stew

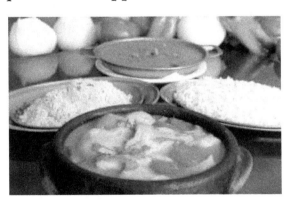

Preparation time: 10 minutes

Cooking time: 20 minutes

Servings: 4

Ingredients:

- 1 pound squash, peeled and roughly cubed
- 1 cup low-sodium chicken stock
- 1 cup canned tomatoes, no-salt-added, crushed
- 1 tablespoon olive oil
- 1 red onion, chopped
- 2 orange sweet peppers, chopped

- 1/2 cup quinoa
- 1/2 tablespoon chives, chopped

Directions:

1. Heat up a pot with the oil over medium heat; add the onion, stir and sauté for 2 minutes.
2. Add the squash and the other ingredients bring to a simmer, and cook for 15 minutes.
3. Stir the stew, divide into bowls and serve for lunch.

Nutrition: 156 calories, 5.8g protein, 23.7g carbohydrates, 5.2g fat, 4.3g fiber, 0mg cholesterol, 52mg sodium, 601mg potassium

Beef And Cabbage Stew

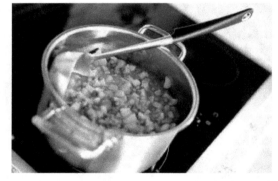

Preparation time: 10 minutes

Cooking time: 20 minutes

Servings: 4

Ingredients:

- 1 green cabbage head, shredded
- 1/4 cup low-sodium beef stock
- 2 tomatoes, cubed
- 2 yellow onions, chopped
- ¾ cup red bell peppers, chopped
- 1 tablespoon olive oil
- 1 pound beef, ground
- 1/4 cup cilantro, chopped
- 1/4 cup green onions, chopped
- 1/4 teaspoon red pepper, crushed

Directions:

1. Heat up a pan with the oil over medium heat, and then add the meat and the onions, stir and brown for 5 minutes.
2. Add the cabbage and the other ingredients, toss, cook for 15 minutes, divide into bowls and serve for lunch.

Nutrition: 329 calories, 38.4g protein, 20.1g carbohydrates, 11g fat, 6.9g fiber, 101mg cholesterol, 142mg sodium, 1,081mg potassium

Pork Stew

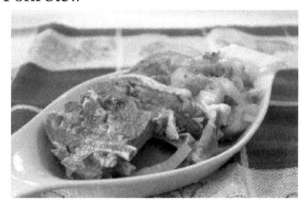

Preparation time: 5 minutes

Cooking time: 8 hours and 10 minutes

Servings: 4

Ingredients:

- 1 pound pork stew meat, cubed
- 1 tablespoon olive oil
- 1/2 pound green beans, trimmed and halved
- 2 yellow onions, chopped
- 2 garlic cloves, minced
- 2 cups low-sodium beef stock
- 8 ounces tomato sauce
- A pinch of black pepper
- A pinch of allspice, ground
- 1 tablespoon rosemary, chopped

Directions:

1. Heat up a pan with the oil over medium-high heat, add the meat, garlic and onion, stir and brown for 10 minutes.
2. Transfer this to a slow cooker, add the other ingredients as well, put the lid on and cook on Low for 8 hours.
3. Divide the stew into bowls and serve.

Nutrition: 357 calories, 38g protein, 16.9g carbohydrates, 14.8g fat, 6.2g fiber, 98mg cholesterol, 587mg sodium, 1,139mg potassium

CHAPTER 6:

Snack

Egg Rolls In A Bowl

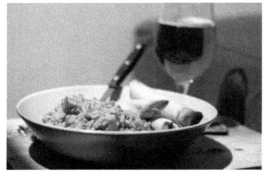

Preparation time: 5 minutes

Cooking Time: 12 minutes

Servings: 4

Ingredients:

- 1 tablespoon olive oil
- A small onion
- 2 cloves garlic
- 1 bag coleslaw mix
- 1/4 cup cilantro leaves for garnish
- 1 pound ground pork or beef
- 1/2 cup beef or chicken stock
- 1 inch ginger sprig, grated
- 1 cup shredded carrots

Sauce Ingredients:

- 1/4 cup gluten-free soy sauce
- 1/4 cup dry sherry
- 1/2 teaspoon black pepper

- 1 tablespoon corn starch
- 2 teaspoons sesame oil
- 1 teaspoon fish sauce

Directions:

1. Brown onions and pork in olive oil and sauté it, adjusting to medium heat. Cook for 2-3 minutes.

2. Add in the broth and onions.

3. Adjust it for 4 minutes, quick release cooking. Add in garlic and ginger, and then sauté, then add shredded veggies, and then cook veggies for 2-3 minutes if you want it softer.

Nutrition: Calories: 440, Fat: 30g, Carbs: 17g, Net Carbs: 13g, Protein: 22g, Fiber: 4g

Instant Pot Quinoa

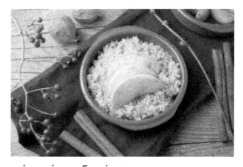

Preparation time: 5 minutes

Cooking Time: 16 minutes

Servings: 6

Ingredients:

- 1 tablespoon avocado oil

- 1 teaspoon minced garlic
- Salt and pepper for taste
- 2 cups quinoa
- 1 diced onion
- 3 cups vegetable broth

Directions:

1. Soak the quinoa in water for about an hour. Put it in mesh strainer and rinse for 3-5 minutes until water is clear.
2. Turn instant pot to sauté.
3. Add onion and oil and cook for 8 minutes. Add in garlic and quinoa, and sauté for 5 minutes, stirring a lot.
4. Add the vegetable broth and salt and pepper, putting lid on the pot, and make sure it's not set to vent.
5. Cook on high pressure for a minute.
6. Do natural pressures release.
7. Remove lid and then serve!

Nutrition: Calories: 240, Fat: 5g, Carbs: 39g, Net Carbs: 35g, Protein: 8g, Fiber: 4g

Instant Pot Pizza Bread

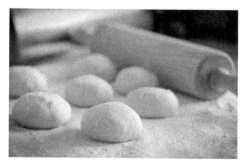

Preparation time: 5 minutes

Cooking Time: 10 minutes

Servings: 4-6

Ingredients:

- 2 cans pizza dough

- 2 cups mozzarella cheese
- 4 cloves minced garlic
- pizza sauce for dipping
- 1/3 cup olive oil
- 2 tablespoons chopped parsley
- 1 pack mini pepperonis

Directions:

1. Cut the dough into 1-inch strips, and then about 1-2 sections.
2. Combine ingredients into bowl, using hands to toss.
3. Put the ingredients in springform or Bundt pan.
4. Add water to bottom, put pan in, and then cook manual on high for 10 minutes, quick release. Let cool then serve.

Nutrition: Calories: 300, Fat: 22g, Carbs: 23g, Net Carbs: 21g, Protein: 18g, Fiber: 2g

Pork Beef Bean Nachos

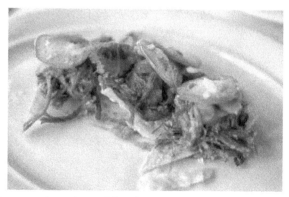

Preparation time: 15 minutes

Cooking Time: 40 minutes

Servings: 10

Ingredients:

- 1 package beef jerky

- 4 cans black beans, drained and rinsed

- 6 bacon strips, crumbled

- 3 pounds pork spareribs

- 1 cup chopped onion

- 4 teaspoons minced garlic

- 4 cups divided beef broth

- Optional toppings such as cheddar, sour cream, green onions, jalapeno slices

- 1 teaspoon crushed red pepper flakes

- Tortilla chips

Directions:

1. Pulse jerky in processor till ground, working in batches, put the ribs in the instant pot, topping with half jerky, two beans, and 1/2 cup onion, three pieces of bacon, 2 teaspoons garlic, 2 cups broth, and half teaspoon red pepper flakes. Cook on high for forty minutes.

2. Let it natural pressure release for 10 minutes, then quick release what's next, and do the same with the second batch.

3. Discard bones, and shred meat and then sauté it, and strain the mixture, and then discard juice and serve with chips and your desired toppings.

Nutrition: Calories: 469, Fat: 24g, Carbs: 27g Net Carbs: 20g, Protein: 33g, Fiber: 7g

Pressure Cooker Cranberry Hot Wings

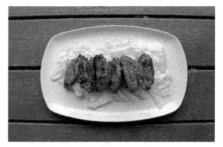

Preparation time: 45 minutes

Cooking Time: 35 minutes

Servings: 4 dozen

Ingredients:

- 1 can jellied cranberry sauce

- 1/4 cup Louisiana-style hot sauce

- 2 tablespoons honey

- 1 tablespoon Dijon mustard

- 1/2 cup sugar-free orange juice

- 2 tablespoons soy sauce

- 2 teaspoons garlic powder

- 1 minced garlic clove

- 1 teaspoon dried minced onion

- 5 pounds chicken wings

- 1 teaspoon salt

- 2 tablespoons cold water

- 4 teaspoons cornstarch

Directions:

1. Whisk the ingredients together, but discard wing tips.

2. Put the wins in your instant pot, and then put cranberry mixture over top.

3. Lock lid, and then adjust pressure to high for 10 minutes.

4. You can from there, do a natural pressure release, and quick pressure.

5. Preheat broiler, skim fat, and from there, let it broil for 20-25 minutes.

6. When browned, brush with the glaze before serving

Nutrition: Calories: 71 per piece, Fat: 4g, Carbs: 5g, Net Carbs: 5g, Protein: 5g, Fiber: 0g

Bacon Hot Dog Bites

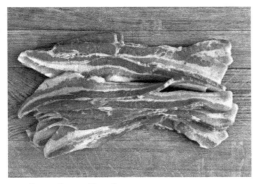

Preparation time: 5 minutes

Cooking Time: 10 minutes

Servings: 12

Ingredients:

- 1 pack of hot dogs
- 1/2 bottle cocktail sauce
- 4 slices smoked bacon

Directions:

1. Cut up the meat, putting the dogs aside and cook bacon till done.

2. Separate the bacon from grease and put the hot dogs and bacon in pot, and then add the cocktail sauce until hated, and then cook on high pressure 5 minutes, then do a quick release.

3. Turn off cooker and put in serving dish, it'll thicken over time.

Nutrition: Calories: 83, Fat: 10g, Carbs: 2g, Net Carbs: 2g, Protein: 10g, Fiber: 0g

Instant Pot Cocktail Wieners

Preparation time: 2 minutes

Cooking Time: 1 min

Servings: 12

Ingredients:

- 1 package 12 cocktail wieners
- 1/4 teaspoon brown sugar
- 1/2 cup chicken or veggie broth
- 1 jar jalapeno jelly
- 1/4 cup chili sauce
- 1 diced jalapeno

Directions:

1. Put 1/2 cup of chicken broth into instant pot, then add wieners and rest of ingredients, still till everything is coated.

2. Cook on high pressure for a minute, and do a quick pressure then serve!

Nutrition: Calories: 92, Fat: 5g, Carbs: 6g, Net Carbs: 5g, Protein: 10g, Fiber: 1g

Pressure Cooker Braised Pulled Ham

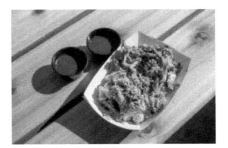

Preparation time: 10 minutes

Cooking Time: 25 minutes

Servings: 16

Ingredients:

- 2 bottles beer, or nonalcoholic beer

- 1/2 teaspoon coarse ground pepper
- 1 cup Dijon mustard, divided
- 1 cooked bone-in ham
- 16 split pretzel hamburger buns
- 4 rosemary sprigs
- Dill pickle slices

Directions:

1. Whisk the beer, pepper and mustard, and then add ham and rosemary, lock lid, and set pressure to high for 20 minutes, then do a natural pressure release.
2. Let it cool, discard rosemary, and skim the fat, and then let it boil for 5 minutes.
3. When ham is cool, shred with forks, discard bone, heat it again, and then put the ham on the pretzel buns, adding Dijon mustard at the end and the dill pickle slices.

Nutrition: Calories: 378, Fat: 9g, Carbs: 50g, Net Carbs: 2g, Protein: 25g, Fiber: 2g

Mini Teriyaki Turkey Sandwiches

Preparation time: 20 minutes

Cooking Time: 30 minutes

Servings: 20

Ingredients:

- 2 chicken breast halves
- 1 cup soy sauce, low-salt
- 1/4 cup cider vinegar
- 3 minced garlic cloves
- 1 tablespoon fresh ginger root
- 2 tablespoons cornstarch
- 20 Hawaiian sweet rolls

- 1/2 teaspoon pepper
- 2 tablespoons melted butter

Directions:

1. Put turkey in pressure cooker and combine the first six ingredients over it.
2. Cook it on manual for 25 minutes, and when finished, natural pressure release. Push sauté after removing the turkey, then mix cornstarch and water, stirring into cooking juices, and cook until sauce is thickened. Shred meat and stir to heat.
3. You can split the rolls, buttering each side, and bake till golden brown, adding the meat mixture to the top.

Nutrition: Calories: 252, Fat: 5g, Carbs: 25g, Net Carbs: 24g, Protein: 26g, Fiber: 1g

Hoisin Meatballs

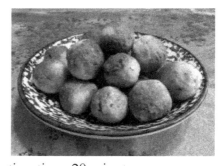

Preparation time: 20 minutes

Cooking Time: 10 minutes

Servings: 2 dozen

Ingredients:

- 1 cup dry red wine or beef broth of choice
- 2 tablespoons soy sauce
- 4 chopped green onions
- 1/4 cup minced cilantro

- 1/4 cup chopped onion
- 1 lightly beaten egg
- 3 tablespoons hoisin sauce
- 2 minced garlic cloves
- 1/2 teaspoon salt and pepper each
- 1 pound ground beef
- 1 pound ground pork of choice
- Sesame seeds for topping

Directions:

1. In instant pot, put the wine, sauces, and boil them, then reduce heat.
2. Combine next 7 ingredients in bowl, then mix it together with the meats, shaping into meatballs, and then put it in instant pot.
3. Set it to manual high pressure for 10 minutes, quick release, and then top with sesame seeds.

Nutrition: Calories: 78, Fat: 5g, Carbs: 1g, Net Carbs: 1g, Protein: 6g, Fiber: 0g

Cuban Pulled Pork Sandwiches

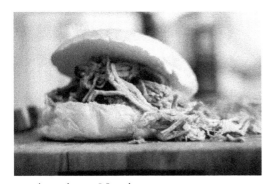

Preparation time: 20 minutes

Cooking Time: 25 minutes

Servings: 16

Ingredients:

- 1 boneless pork shoulder butt roast

- 2 teaspoons salt and pepper
- 1 cup orange juice
- 1/2 cup lime juice
- 1 tablespoon olive oil
- 12 minced garlic cloves
- 2 tablespoons ground coriander
- 1 teaspoon cayenne pepper
- 2 teaspoons white pepper

For the sandwiches:

- 2 loaves French bread
- 16 dill pickle slices
- 1 pound sliced Swiss cheese
- 1 pound sliced deli ham
- Mustard for topping

Directions:

1. Cut pork into small, 2 inch pieces, and season with salt and pepper, then brown it in the instant pot after turning it onto sauté.
2. Add in the juices, and scrape the brown bits, then add the garlic, coriander, white pepper, and the cayenne pepper, and then put pork in there, and then cook it on manual high pressure for 25 minutes.
3. When finished, do a natural pressure release, and then quick release it, and then shred with forks, and then remove a cup of the liquid, and then toss this together.
4. Prepare sandwiches with the bread halves, then pickles, ham, pork, cheese, and then the tops.

Nutrition: Calories: 573, Fat: 28g, Carbs: 35g, Net Carbs: 33g, Protein: 45g, Fiber: 2g

Instant Pot Polenta

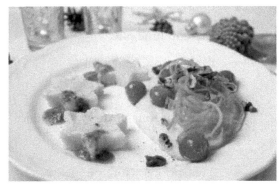

Preparation time: 5 minutes

Cooking Time: 25 minutes

Serves: 5

Ingredients:

- 4 cups veggie broth of water
- Black pepper for taste
- 2 teaspoons salt
- 1 teaspoon onion powder
- 1 teaspoon granulated garlic powder
- 1 teaspoon dried herb mix
- 1 cup cornmeal

Directions:

1. Turn IP to sauté, then add the water, salt, spices, and herbs, and then let it simmer for 5 minutes.

2. Stir in cornmeal for a minute till the limps are gone.

3. Let it cook for 8 minutes on high and then do a natural pressure release.

4. Swirl in your choice of butter or cheese, and then serve it.

Nutrition: Calories: 130, Fat: 6g, Carbs: 3g, Net Carbs: 3g, Protein: 5g, Fiber: 3g

Asian Glazed Meatballs

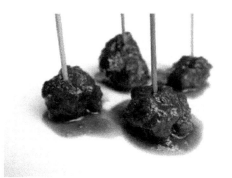

Preparation time: 20 minutes

Cooking Time: 20 minutes

Servings: 6

Ingredients:

- 2 room temperature eggs
- 4 chopped green onions
- 2 tablespoons minced ginger
- 2 teaspoons sesame oil
- 1/2 teaspoon black pepper and salt to taste
- 1 cup GF panko breadcrumbs
- 3 cloves minced garlic
- 2 tablespoons Tamari
- Chili flake sand sriracha to taste
- 3 tablespoons apple cider vinegar
- 1/3 cup honey
- 1 teaspoon grated ginger
- 1 cup hoisin sauce

Directions:

1. Combine eggs, crumbs, green onions, ginger, sauce, and rest of ingredients, thoroughly mixing with hands to make meatballs.

2. Take the glaze ingredients and sauté them in instant pot for 3-4 minutes to simmer.

3. Add 2 tablespoons of olive oil to instant pot, and sauté them for 2 minutes each side, and then cover and cook on manual for 10 minutes.

4. Do a natural pressure release, and then coat with glaze, and top with sesame seeds and reserved onions.

Nutrition: Calories: 217, Fat: 4g, Carbs: 39g, Net Carbs: 38g, Protein: 5g, Fiber: 1g

Jalapeno Cheddar Cornbread

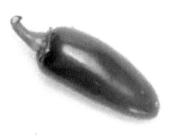

Preparation time: 5 minutes

Cooking Time: 25 minutes

Servings: 12

Ingredients:

- A box of cornbread mix
- 1 cup milk
- 1/4 cup scallions
- 1/2 cup pickled jalapeno, chopped
- 1/2 cup shredded cheddar cheese
- 1 egg
- 1/4 cup olive oil
- 1/4 cup corn
- 2 cups shredded cheddar cheese

Directions:

1. Mix the wet ingredients together till incorporated, and then from there add the scallions, corn, jalapenos, and shredded cheese, then fold into the batter.

2. Line tray with cupcake liners and add the mixtures, and from there, put it in the instant pot, cooking on high pressure for 25 minutes.

3. Use a natural pressure release, and then serve them.

Nutrition: Calories: 283, Fat: 16g, Carbs: 26g, Net Carbs: 24g, Protein: 8g, Fiber: 2g

CHAPTER 7:

Side Dishes

Zucchini And Brussels Sprouts Salad

Preparation time: 10 minutes

Cooking time: 3 hours

Servings: 4

Ingredients:

- 1 pound zucchinis, roughly cubed

- 1/2 pound Brussels sprouts, trimmed and halved

- 1/4 cup veggie stock, low-sodium

- 1 teaspoon cumin, ground

- 1 teaspoon chili powder

- 2 teaspoons avocado oil

Directions:

1. In slow cooker, combine the sprouts with the zucchinis and the other ingredients, put the lid on and cook it on Low for three hours.

2. Divide between plates and serve as a side dish.

Nutrition: Calories 51, Fat 0.9g, Cholesterol 0mg, Sodium 42mg, Carbohydrate 9.8g, Fiber 3.8g, Sugars 3.3g, Protein 3.5g, Potassium 547mg

Spiced Broccoli Florets

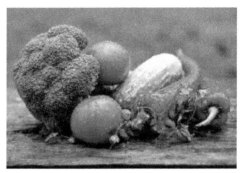

Preparation time: 10 minutes

Cooking time: 3 hours

Servings: 10

Ingredients:

- 6 cups broccoli florets

- 1 and 1/2 cups low-fat cheddar cheese, shredded

- 1/2 teaspoon cider vinegar

- 1/4 cup yellow onion, chopped

- 10 ounces tomato sauce, sodium-free

- 2 tablespoons olive oil

- A pinch of black pepper

Directions:

1. Grease your slow cooker with the oil, add broccoli, tomato sauce, cider vinegar, onion and black pepper, cover and cook on High for 2 hours and 30 minutes.

2. Sprinkle the cheese all over, cover, cook on High for 30 minutes more, divide between plates and serve as a side dish.

Nutrition: Calories 119, Fat 8.7g, Cholesterol 18mg, Sodium 272mg, Carbohydrate 5.7g, Fiber 1.9g, Sugars 2.3g, Protein 6.2g, Potassium 288mg

Lima Beans Dish

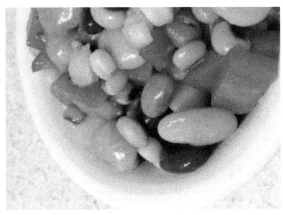

Preparation time: 10 minutes

Cooking time: 5 hours

Servings: 10

Ingredients:

- 1 green bell pepper, chopped

- 1 sweet red pepper, chopped

- 1 and 1/2 cups tomato sauce, salt-free

- 1 yellow onion, chopped

- 1/2 cup water

- 16 ounces canned kidney beans, no-salt-added, drained and rinsed

- 16 ounces canned black-eyed peas, no-salt-added, drained and rinsed

- 15 ounces corn

- 15 ounces canned lima beans, no-salt-added, drained and rinsed

- 15 ounces canned black beans, no-salt-added, drained and rinsed

- 2 celery ribs, chopped

- 2 bay leaves

- 1 teaspoon ground mustard

- 1 tablespoon cider vinegar

Directions:

1. In your slow cooker, mix the tomato sauce with the onion, celery, red pepper, green bell pepper, water, bay leaves, mustard, vinegar, kidney beans, black-eyed peas, corn, lima beans and black beans, cover and cook on Low for 5 hours.

2. Discard bay leaves, divide the whole mix between plates and serve.

Nutrition: Calories 602, Fat 4.8g, Cholesterol 0mg, Sodium 255mg, Carbohydrate 117.7g, Fiber 24.6g, Sugars 13.4g, Protein 33g, Potassium 2355mg

Soy Sauce Green Beans

Preparation time: 10 minutes

Cooking time: 2 hours

Servings: 12

Ingredients:

- 3 tablespoons olive oil

- 16 ounces green beans

- 1/2 teaspoon garlic powder

- 1/2 cup coconut sugar

- 1 teaspoon low-sodium soy sauce

Directions:

1. In your slow cooker, mix the green beans with the oil, sugar, soy sauce and garlic powder, cover and cook on Low for 2 hours.

2. Toss the beans, divide them between plates and serve as a side dish.

Nutrition: Calories 46, Fat 3.6g, Cholesterol 0mg, Sodium 29mg, Carbohydrate 3.6g, Fiber 1.3g, Sugars 0.6g, Protein 0.8g, Potassium 80mg

Butter Corn

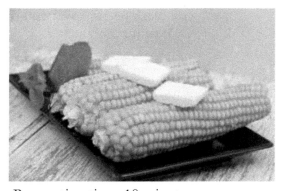

Preparation time: 10 minutes

Cooking time: 4 hours

Servings: 12

Ingredients:

- 20 ounces fat-free cream cheese

- 10 cups corn

- 1/2 cup low-fat butter

- 1/2 cup fat-free milk

- A pinch of black pepper

- 2 tablespoons green onions, chopped

Directions:

1. In your slow cooker, mix the corn with cream cheese, milk, butter, black pepper and onions, toss, cover and cook on Low for 4 hours.

2. Toss one more time, divide between plates and serve as a side dish.

Nutrition: Calories 279, Fat 18g, Cholesterol 52mg, Sodium 165mg, Carbohydrate 26g, Fiber 3.5g, Sugars 4.8g, Protein 8.1g, Potassium 422mg

Stevia Peas With Marjoram

Preparation time: 10 minutes

Cooking time: 5 hours

Servings: 12

Ingredients:

- 1 pound carrots, sliced

- 1 yellow onion, chopped

- 16 ounces peas

- 2 tablespoons stevia

- 2 tablespoons olive oil

- 4 garlic cloves, minced

- 1/4 cup water

- 1 teaspoon marjoram, dried

- A pinch of white pepper

Directions:

1. In your slow cooker, mix the carrots with water, onion, oil, stevia, garlic, marjoram, white pepper and peas, toss, cover and cook on High for 5 hours.

2. Divide between plates and serve as a side dish.

Nutrition: Calories 71, Fat 2.5g, Cholesterol 0mg, Sodium 29mg, Carbohydrate 12.1g, Fiber 3.1g, Sugars 4.4g, Protein 2.5g, Potassium 231mg

Pilaf With Bella Mushrooms

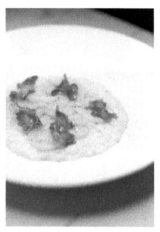

Preparation time: 10 minutes

Cooking time: 3 hours

Servings: 6

Ingredients:

- 1 cup wild rice

- 6 green onions, chopped

- 1/2 pound baby Bella mushrooms

- 2 cups water

- 2 tablespoons olive oil

- 2 garlic cloves, minced

Directions:

1. In your slow cooker, mix the rice with garlic, onions, oil, mushrooms and water, toss, cover and cook on Low for 3 hours.

2. Stir the pilaf one more time, divide between plates and serve.

Nutrition: Calories 151, Fat 5.1g, Cholesterol 0mg, Sodium 9mg, Carbohydrate 23.3g, Fiber 2.6g, Sugars 1.7g, Protein 5.2g, Potassium 343mg

Parsley Fennel

Preparation time: 10 minutes

Cooking time: 2 hours and 30 minutes

Servings: 4

Ingredients:

- 2 fennel bulbs, sliced

- Juice and zest of 1 lime

- 2 teaspoons avocado oil

- 1/2 teaspoon turmeric powder

- 1 tablespoon parsley, chopped

- 1/4 cup veggie stock, low-sodium

Directions:

1. In slow cooker, combine the fennel with the lime juice, zest and the other ingredients, put the lid on and cook on Low for 2 hours and 30 minutes.

2. Divide between plates and serve as a side dish.

Nutrition: Calories 47, Fat 0.6g, Cholesterol 0mg, Sodium 71mg, Carbohydrate 10.8g, Fiber 4.3g, Sugars 0.4g, Protein 1.7g, Potassium 521mg

Sweet Butternut

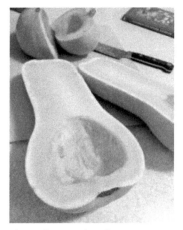

Preparation time: 10 minutes

Cooking time: 4 hours

Servings: 8

Ingredients:

- 1 cup carrots, chopped
- 1 tablespoon olive oil
- 1 yellow onion, chopped
- 1/2 teaspoon stevia
- 1 garlic clove, minced
- 1/2 teaspoon curry powder
- 1 butternut squash, cubed
- 2 and 1/2 cups low-sodium veggie stock
- 1/2 cup basmati rice
- ¾ cup coconut milk
- 1/2 teaspoon cinnamon powder
- 1/4 teaspoon ginger, grated

Directions:

1. Heat up a pan with the oil over medium-high heat, add the oil, onion, garlic, stevia, carrots, curry powder, cinnamon and ginger, stir, cook for 5 minutes and transfer to your slow cooker.

2. Add squash, stock and coconut milk, stir, cover and cook on Low for 4 hours.

3. Divide the butternut mix between plates and serve as a side dish.

Nutrition: Calories 134, Fat 7.2g, Cholesterol 0mg, Sodium 59mg, Carbohydrate 16.5g, Fiber 1.7g, Sugars 2.7g, Protein 1.8g, Potassium 202mg

Mushroom Sausages

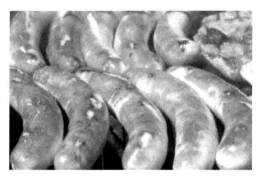

Preparation time: 10 minutes

Cooking time: 2 hours

Servings: 12

Ingredients:

- 6 celery ribs, chopped
- 1 pound no-sugar, beef sausage, chopped
- 2 tablespoons olive oil
- 1/2 pound mushrooms, chopped
- 1/2 cup sunflower seeds, peeled
- 1 cup low-sodium veggie stock
- 1 cup cranberries, dried
- 2 yellow onions, chopped
- 2 garlic cloves, minced

- 1 tablespoon sage, dried

- 1 whole wheat bread loaf, cubed

Directions:

1. Heat up a pan with the oil over medium- high heat, add beef, stir and brown for a few minutes.

2. Add mushrooms, onion, celery, garlic and sage, stir, cook for a few more minutes and transfer to your slow cooker.

3. Add stock, cranberries, sunflower seeds and the bread cubes, cover and cook on High for 2 hours. Stir the whole mix, divide between plates and serve as a side dish.

Nutrition: Calories 188, Fat 13.8g, Cholesterol 25mg, Sodium 489mg, Carbohydrate 8.2g, Fiber 1.9g, Sugars 2.2g, Protein 7.6g, Potassium 254mg

Parsley Red Potatoes

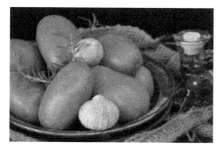

Preparation time: 10 minutes

Cooking time: 6 hours

Servings: 8

Ingredients:

- 16 baby red potatoes, halved

- 2 cups low-sodium chicken stock

- 1 carrot, sliced

- 1 celery rib, chopped

- 1/4 cup yellow onion, chopped

- 1 tablespoon parsley, chopped

- 2 tablespoons olive oil

- A pinch of black pepper

- 1 garlic clove minced

Directions:

1. In your slow cooker, mix the potatoes with the carrot, celery, onion, stock, parsley, garlic, oil and black pepper, toss, cover and cook on Low for 6 hours.

2. Divide between plates and serve as a side dish.

Nutrition: Calories 257, Fat 9.5g, Cholesterol 0mg, Sodium 845mg, Carbohydrate 43.4g, Fiber 4.4g, Sugars 4.6g, Protein 4.4g, Potassium 47mg

Jalapeno Black-Eyed Peas Mix

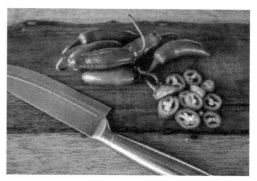

Preparation time: 10 minutes

Cooking time: 5 hours

Servings: 12

Ingredients:

- 17 ounces black-eyed peas

- 1 sweet red pepper, chopped

- 1/2 cup sausage, chopped

- 1 yellow onion, chopped
- 1 jalapeno, chopped
- 2 garlic cloves minced
- 6 cups water
- 1/2 teaspoon cumin, ground
- A pinch of black pepper
- 2 tablespoons cilantro, chopped

Directions:

1. In your slow cooker, mix the peas with the sausage, onion, red pepper, jalapeno, garlic, cumin, black pepper, water and cilantro, cover and cook on Low for 5 hours.

2. Divide between plates and serve as a side dish.

Nutrition: Calories 75, Fat 3.5g, Cholesterol 9mg, Sodium 94mg, Carbohydrate 7.2g, Fiber 1.7g, Sugars 0.9g, Protein 4.3g, Potassium 142mg

Sour Cream Green Beans

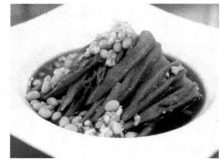

Preparation time: 10 minutes

Cooking time: 4 hours

Servings: 8

Ingredients:

- 15 ounces green beans
- 14 ounces corn

- 4 ounces mushrooms, sliced
- 11 ounces cream of mushroom soup, low-fat and sodium-free
- 1/2 cup low-fat sour cream
- 1/2 cup almonds, chopped
- 1/2 cup low-fat cheddar cheese, shredded

Directions:

1. In your slow cooker, mix the green beans with the corn, mushrooms soup, mushrooms, almonds, cheese and sour cream, toss, cover and cook on Low for 4 hours.

2. Stir one more time, divide between plates and serve as a side dish.

Nutrition: Calories360, Fat 12.7g, Cholesterol 14mg, Sodium 220mg, Carbohydrate 58.3g, Fiber 10g, Sugars 10.3g, Protein 14g, Potassium 967mg

Cumin Brussels Sprouts

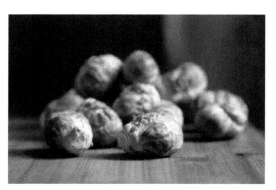

Preparation time: 10 minutes

Cooking time: 3 hours

Servings: 4

Ingredients:

- 1 cup low-sodium veggie stock

- 1 pound Brussels sprouts, trimmed and halved
- 1 teaspoon rosemary, dried
- 1 teaspoon cumin, ground
- 1 tablespoon mint, chopped

Directions:

1. In your slow cooker, combine the sprouts with the stock and the other ingredients, put the lid on and cook on Low for 3 hours.
2. Divide between plates and serve as a side dish.

Nutrition: Calories 56, Fat 0.6g, Cholesterol 0mg, Sodium 65mg, Carbohydrate 11.4g, Fiber 4.5g, Sugars 2.7g, Protein 4g, Potassium 460mg

Peach And Carrots

Preparation time: 10 minutes

Cooking time: 6 hours

Servings: 6

Ingredients:

- 2 pounds small carrots, peeled
- 1/2 cup low-fat butter, melted
- 1/2 cup canned peach, unsweetened
- 2 tablespoons cornstarch
- 3 tablespoons stevia
- 2 tablespoons water
- 1/2 teaspoon cinnamon powder
- 1 teaspoon vanilla extract
- A pinch of nutmeg, ground

Directions:

1. In your slow cooker, mix the carrots with the butter, peach, stevia, cinnamon, vanilla, nutmeg and cornstarch mixed with water, toss, cover and cook on Low for 6 hours.
2. Toss the carrots one more time, divide between plates and serve as a side dish.

Nutrition: Calories139, Fat 10.7g, Cholesterol 0mg, Sodium 199mg, Carbohydrate 35.4g, Fiber 4.2g, Sugars 6.9g, Protein 3.8g, Potassium 25mg

Baby Spinach And Grains Mix

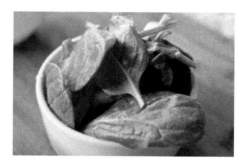

Preparation time: 10 minutes

Cooking time: 4 hours

Servings: 12

Ingredients:

- 1 butternut squash, peeled and cubed
- 1 cup whole grain blend, uncooked
- 12 ounces low-sodium veggie stock
- 6 ounces baby spinach
- 1 yellow onion, chopped
- 3 garlic cloves, minced

- 1/2 cup water

- 2 teaspoons thyme, chopped

- A pinch of black pepper

Directions:

1. In your slow cooker, mix the squash with whole grain, onion, garlic, water, thyme, black pepper, stock and spinach, cover and cook on Low for 4 hours.

2. Divide between plates and serve as a side dish.

Nutrition: Calories78, Fat 0.6g, Cholesterol 0mg, Sodium 259mg, Carbohydrate 16.4g, Fiber 1.8g, Sugars 2g, Protein 2.5g, Potassium 138mg

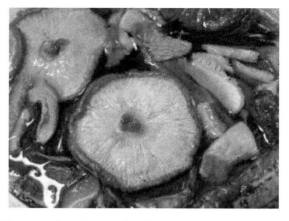

Preparation time: 10 minutes

Cooking time: 4 hours

Servings: 6

Ingredients:

- 1 pound mushrooms, halved

- 1 teaspoon Italian seasoning

- 3 tablespoons olive oil

- 1 cup tomato sauce, no-salt-added

- 1 yellow onion, chopped

Directions:

1. In your slow cooker, mix the mushrooms with the oil, onion, Italian seasoning and tomato sauce, toss, cover and cook on Low for 4 hours.

2. Divide between plates and serve as a side dish.

Nutrition: Calories96, Fat 7.5g, Cholesterol 1mg, Sodium 219mg, Carbohydrate 6.5g, Fiber 1.8g, Sugars 3.9g, Protein 3.1g, Potassium 403mg

Italians Style Mushroom Mix

CHAPTER 8:

Soups and Stews

Golden Mushroom Soup

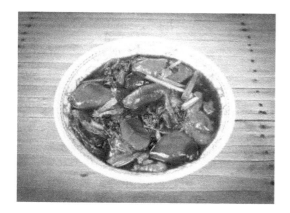

Preparation Time: 10 MINUTES

Cooking Time: 8 HOURS

Servings: 6

Ingredients:

- 1 onion, finely chopped
- 1 carrot, peeled and finely chopped
- 1 fennel bulb, finely chopped
- 1 pound fresh mushrooms, quartered
- 8 cups Vegetable Broth (here), Poultry Broth (here), or store bought
- 1/4 cup dry sherry
- 1 teaspoon dried thyme
- 1 teaspoon garlic powder
- 1/2 teaspoon sea salt
- 1/8 teaspoon freshly ground black pepper

Directions:

1. In your slow cooker, combine all the ingredients, mixing to combine.

2. Cover and set on low. Cook for 8 hours.

NUTRITION: Calories: 71; Total Fat: 0g; Saturated Fat: 0g; Cholesterol: 0mg; Carbohydrates: 15g; Fiber: 3g; Protein: 3g

Minestrone

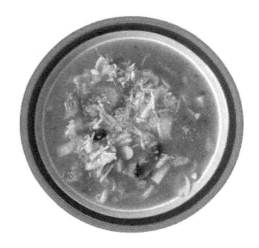

Preparation Time: 15 MINUTES

Cooking Time: 9 HOURS

Servings: 6

Ingredients:

- 2 carrots, peeled and sliced
- 2 celery stalks, sliced
- 1 onion, chopped
- 2 cups green beans, chopped
- 1 (16-ounce) can crushed tomatoes
- 2 cups cooked kidney beans (here), rinsed

- 6 cups Poultry Broth (here), Vegetable Broth (here), or store bought
- 1 teaspoon garlic powder
- 1 teaspoon dried Italian seasoning
- 1/4 teaspoon sea salt
- 1/4 teaspoons freshly ground black pepper
- 11/2 cups cooked whole-wheat elbow macaroni (or pasta shape of your choice)
- 1 zucchini, chopped

Directions:

1. In your slow cooker, combine the carrots, celery, onion, green beans, tomatoes, kidney beans, broth, garlic powder, Italian seasoning, salt, and pepper in the slow cooker.

2. Cover and cook on low for 8 hours.

3. Stir in the macaroni and zucchini. Cover and cook on low for 1 hour more.

NUTRITION: Calories: 193; Total Fat: 0g; Saturated Fat: 0g; Cholesterol: 1mg; Carbohydrates: 39g; Fiber: 10g; Protein: 10g

Pumpkin Soup

Preparation Time: 5 MINUTES

Cooking Time: 8 HOURS

Servings: 6

Ingredients:

- 1 (29-ounce) can pumpkin purée
- 2 carrots, peeled and chopped
- 1 onion, chopped
- 5 cups Vegetable Broth (here), or store bought
- 1 (14-ounce) can light coconut milk
- 1 teaspoon garlic powder
- 1 teaspoon onion powder

- 1 teaspoon ground cumin
- 1/2 teaspoon sea salt
- 1/4 teaspoons freshly ground black pepper
- 3 tablespoons toasted pumpkin seeds (optional)
- 1 tablespoon chopped fresh chives (optional)

Directions:

1. In your slow cooker, combine the pumpkin purée, carrots, onion, broth, coconut milk, garlic powder, onion powder, cumin, salt, and pepper.

2. Cover and cook on low for 8 hours.

3. Purée with an immersion blender.

4. Serve sprinkled with pumpkin seeds and chives, if desired.

NUTRITION: Calories: 264; Total Fat: 18g; Saturated Fat: 14g; Cholesterol: 0mg; Carbohydrates: 24g; Fiber: 6g; Protein: 4g

Lentil Soup

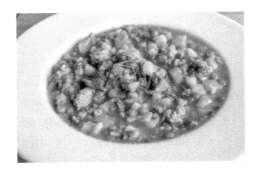

Preparation Time: 10 MINUTES

Cooking Time: 8 HOURS

Servings: 6

Ingredients:

- 1 pound dried lentils, soaked overnight and rinsed

- 3 carrots, peeled and chopped
- 1 celery stalk, chopped
- 1 onion, chopped
- 6 cups Vegetable Broth (here), Poultry Broth (here), Beef Broth (here), or store bought
- 11/2 teaspoons garlic powder
- 1 teaspoon ground cumin
- 1 teaspoon smoked paprika
- 1 teaspoon dried thyme
- 1/4 teaspoon liquid smoke
- 1/4 teaspoon sea salt
- 1/4 teaspoons freshly ground black pepper

Directions:

1. In your slow cooker, combine the lentils with all the other ingredients.

2. Cover and cook on low for 8 hours. Stir and serve.

NUTRITION: Calories: 307; Total Fat: 1g; Saturated Fat: 0g; Cholesterol: 0mg; Carbohydrates: 56g; Fiber: 25g; Protein: 20g

Black Bean Soup

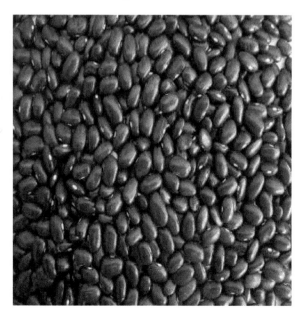

Preparation Time: 10 MINUTES

Cooking Time: 8 HOURS

Servings: 6

Ingredients:

- 1 pound dried black beans, soaked overnight and rinsed
- 1 onion, chopped
- 1 carrot, peeled and chopped
- 2 jalapeño peppers, seeded and diced
- 6 cups Vegetable Broth (here), or store bought
- 1 teaspoon ground cumin
- 1 teaspoon ground coriander
- 1 teaspoon chili powder
- 1/2 teaspoon ground chipotle pepper (or more to taste)
- 1/2 teaspoon sea salt
- 1/4 teaspoons freshly ground black pepper
- Pinch cayenne pepper
- 1/4 cup fat-free sour cream, for garnish (optional)
- 1/4 cup grated low-fat Cheddar cheese, for garnish (optional)

Directions:

1. In your slow cooker, combine all the ingredients.

2. Cover and cook on low for 8 hours.

3. If you'd like, mash the beans with a potato masher, or purée using an immersion blender, blender, or food processor.

4. Serve topped with the optional garnishes, if desired.

NUTRITION: Calories: 320; Total Fat: 3g; Saturated Fat: 1g; Cholesterol: 6mg; Carbohydrates: 57g; Fiber: 13g; Protein: 18g

Chickpea & Kale Soup

Preparation Time: 10 MINUTES

Cooking Time: 9 HOURS

Servings: 6

Ingredients:

- 1 summer squash, quartered lengthwise and sliced crosswise
- 1 zucchini, quartered lengthwise and sliced crosswise
- 2 cups cooked chickpeas (here), rinsed
- 1 cup uncooked quinoa
- 2 (14-ounce) cans diced tomatoes, with their juice
- 5 cups Vegetable Broth (here), Poultry Broth (here), or store bought
- 1 teaspoon garlic powder
- 1 teaspoon onion powder
- 1 teaspoon dried thyme
- 1/2 teaspoon sea salt
- 2 cups chopped kale leaves

Directions:

1. In your slow cooker, combine the summer squash, zucchini, chickpeas, quinoa, tomatoes (with their juice), broth, garlic powder, onion powder, thyme, and salt.

2. Cover and cook on low for 8 hours.

3. Stir in the kale. Cover and cook on low for 1 more hour.

NUTRITION: Calories: 221; Total Fat: 3g; Saturated Fat: 0g; Cholesterol: 0mg; Carbohydrates: 40g; Fiber: 7g; Protein: 10g

Clam Chowder

Preparation Time: 15 MINUTES

Cooking Time: 8 HOURS

Servings: 6

Ingredients:

- 1 red onion, chopped
- 3 carrots, peeled and chopped
- 1 fennel bulb and fronds, chopped
- 1 (10-ounce) can chopped clams, with their juice
- 1 pound baby red potatoes, quartered
- 4 cups Poultry Broth (here), or store bought
- 1/2 teaspoon sea salt
- 1/8 teaspoon freshly ground black pepper
- 2 cups skim milk
- 1/4 pound turkey bacon, browned and crumbled, for garnish

Directions:

1. In your slow cooker, combine the onion, carrots, fennel bulb and fronds, clams (with their juice), potatoes, broth, salt, and pepper.

2. Cover and cook on low for 8 hours.

3. Stir in the milk and serve garnished with the crumbled bacon.

NUTRITION: Calories: 172; Total Fat: 1g; Saturated Fat: 0g; Cholesterol: 14mg; Carbohydrates: 29g; Fiber: 4g; Protein: 10g

Chicken & Rice Soup

Preparation Time: 10 MINUTES

Cooking Time: 8 HOURS

Servings: 6

Ingredients:

- 1 pound boneless, skinless chicken thighs, cut into 1-inch pieces
- 1 onion, chopped
- 3 carrots, peeled and sliced
- 2 celery stalks, sliced
- 6 cups Poultry Broth (here), or store bought
- 1 teaspoon garlic powder
- 1 teaspoon dried rosemary
- 1/4 teaspoon sea salt
- 1/4 teaspoons freshly ground black pepper
- 3 cups cooked Brown Rice (here)

Directions:

1. In your slow cooker, combine the chicken, onion, carrots, celery, broth, garlic powder, rosemary, salt, and pepper.

2. Cover and cook on low for 8 hours.

3. Stir in the rice about 10 minutes before serving, and allow the broth to warm it.

NUTRITION: Calories: 354; Total Fat: 7g; Saturated Fat: 2g; Cholesterol: 67mg; Carbohydrates: 43g; Fiber: 3g; Protein: 28g

Chicken Corn Chowder

Preparation Time: 10 MINUTES

Cooking Time: 8 HOURS

Servings: 6

Ingredients:

- 1 pound boneless, skinless chicken thighs, cut into 1-inch pieces
- 2 onions, chopped
- 3 jalapeño peppers, seeded and minced
- 2 red bell peppers, seeded and chopped
- 11/2 cups fresh or frozen corn
- 6 cups Poultry Broth (here), or store bought
- 1 teaspoon garlic powder
- 1/2 teaspoon sea salt
- 1/4 teaspoons freshly ground black pepper
- 1 cup skim milk

Directions:

1. In your slow cooker, combine the chicken, onions, jalapeños, red bell peppers, corn, broth, garlic powder, salt, and pepper.

2. Cover and cook on low for 8 hours.

3. Stir in the skim milk just before serving.

NUTRITION: Calories: 236; Total Fat: 6g; Saturated Fat: 2g; Cholesterol: 68mg; Carbohydrates: 17g; Fiber: 3g; Protein: 27g

Turkey Ginger Soup

Preparation Time: 10 MINUTES

Cooking Time: 8 HOURS

Servings: 6

Ingredients:

- 1 pound boneless, skinless turkey thighs, cut into 1-inch pieces
- 1 pound fresh shiitake mushrooms, halved
- 3 carrots, peeled and sliced

- 2 cups frozen peas
- 1 tablespoon grated fresh ginger
- 6 cups Poultry Broth (here), or store bought
- 1 tablespoon low-sodium soy sauce
- 1 teaspoon toasted sesame oil
- 2 teaspoons garlic powder
- 11/2 cups cooked Brown Rice (here)

Directions:

1. In your slow cooker, combine the turkey, mushrooms, carrots, peas, ginger, broth, soy sauce, sesame oil, and garlic powder.

2. Cover and cook on low for 8 hours.

3. About 30 minutes before serving, stir in the rice to warm it through.

NUTRITION: Calories: 318; Total Fat: 7g; Saturated Fat: 0g; Cholesterol: 0mg; Carbohydrates: 42g; Fiber: 6g; Protein: 24g

Taco Soup

Preparation Time: 15 MINUTES

Cooking Time: 8 HOURS

Servings: 6

Ingredients:

- 1 pound ground turkey breast
- 1 onion, chopped
- 1 (14-ounce) can tomatoes and green chiles, with their juice
- 6 cups Poultry Broth (here), or store bought
- 1 teaspoon chili powder
- 1 teaspoon ground cumin
- 1/2 teaspoon sea salt
- 1/4 cup chopped fresh cilantro
- Juice of 1 lime

- 1/2 cup grated low-fat Cheddar cheese

Directions:

1. Crumble the turkey into the slow cooker.

2. Add the onion, tomatoes and green chiles (with their juice), broth, chili powder, cumin, and salt.

3. Cover and cook on low for 8 hours.

4. Stir in the cilantro and lime juice.

5. Serve garnished with the cheese.

NUTRITION: Calories: 281; Total Fat: 10g; Saturated Fat: 4g; Cholesterol: 66mg; Carbohydrates: 20g; Fiber: 5g; Protein: 30g

Italian Sausage & Fennel Soup

Preparation Time: 10 MINUTES

Cooking Time: 8 HOURS

Servings: 6

Ingredients:

- 1 pound Italian chicken or turkey sausage, cut into 1/2-inch slices
- 2 onions, chopped
- 1 fennel bulb, chopped
- 6 cups Poultry Broth (here), or store bought
- 1/4 cup dry sherry
- 11/2 teaspoons garlic powder
- 1 teaspoon dried thyme
- 1/2 teaspoon sea salt
- 1/4 teaspoons freshly ground black pepper
- Pinch red pepper flakes

Directions:

1. In your slow cooker, combine all the ingredients.

2.   Cover and cook on low for 8 hours.

NUTRITION: Calories: 311; Total Fat: 22g; Saturated Fat: 7g; Cholesterol: 64mg; Carbohydrates: 8g; Fiber: 2g; Protein: 18g

Pork, Fennel & Apple Stew

Preparation Time: 15 MINUTES

Cooking Time: 8 HOURS

Servings: 6

Ingredients:

- 1 pound pork shoulder, trimmed of as much fat as possible and cut into 1-inch cubes
- 2 sweet-tart apples (such as Braeburn), peeled, cored, and sliced
- 1 fennel bulb, sliced
- 2 red onions, sliced
- 1/4 cup apple cider vinegar
- 2 cups Poultry Broth (here), or store bought
- 1 teaspoon garlic powder
- 1 teaspoon ground mustard
- 1/2 teaspoon ground cinnamon
- 1/2 teaspoon sea salt
- 1/8 teaspoon freshly ground black pepper

Directions:

1.   In your slow cooker, combine all the ingredients.

2.   Cover and cook on low for 8 hours.

NUTRITION: Calories: 297; Total Fat: 11g; Saturated Fat: 4g; Cholesterol: 76mg; Carbohydrates: 15g; Fiber: 4g; Protein: 21g

Vietnamese Beef Stew

Preparation Time: 15 MINUTES

Cooking Time: 8 HOURS

Servings: 6

Ingredients:

- 2 cups Beef Broth (here), or store bought
- 1 tablespoon cornstarch
- 1 pound stew beef, trimmed and cut into 1-inch cubes
- 3 carrots, peeled and chopped
- 1 onion, sliced
- 1 (14-ounce) can crushed tomatoes, with their juice
- 1 tablespoon honey
- 1 teaspoon Asian fish sauce
- 1 tablespoon five-spice powder
- 1 teaspoon garlic powder
- 1/4 teaspoons freshly ground black pepper

Directions:

1.   In a small bowl, whisk together the broth and cornstarch.

2.   Add the mixture to your slow cooker, along with the remaining ingredients.

3.   Cover and cook on low for 8 hours.

NUTRITION: Calories: 187; Total Fat: 5g; Saturated Fat: 0g; Cholesterol: 0mg; Carbohydrates: 15g; Fiber: 4g; Protein: 20g

Sweet Potato Curry With Lentils

Preparation Time: 10 MINUTES

Cooking Time: 8 HOURS

Servings: 4

Ingredients:

- 4 sweet potatoes, peeled and cut into 1-inch cubes
- 1 onion, chopped
- 1 cup dried green lentils, soaked overnight and rinsed
- 1 (14-ounce) can chopped tomatoes, with their juice
- 1 cup canned light coconut milk
- 1 cup Vegetable Broth (here), or store bought
- 1 tablespoon curry powder
- 1 teaspoon garlic powder
- 1/2 teaspoon sea salt
- 2 tablespoons chopped fresh cilantro

Directions:

1. In your slow cooker, combine the sweet potatoes, onion, lentils, tomatoes (with their juice), coconut milk, broth, curry powder, garlic powder, and salt.

2. Cover and cook on low for 8 hours.

3. Stir in the cilantro and serve.

NUTRITION: Calories: 525; Total Fat: 16g; Saturated Fat: 13g; Cholesterol: 0mg; Carbohydrates: 83g; Fiber: 25g; Protein: 18g

CHAPTER 9:

Salads

Seafood Arugula Salad

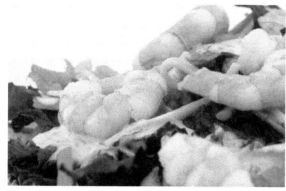

Preparation time: 5 minutes

Cooking time: 10 minutes

Servings: 4

Ingredients:
- 1 tablespoon olive oil
- 2 cups shrimps, cooked
- 1 cup arugula
- 1 tablespoon cilantro, chopped

Directions:
1. Put all ingredients in the salad bowl and shake well.

Nutrition: 61 calories, 6.6g protein, 0.2g carbohydrates, 3.7g fat, 0.1g fiber, 123mg cholesterol, 216mg sodium, 20mg potassium.

Smoked Salad

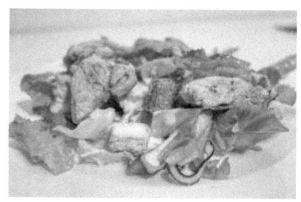

Preparation time: 10 minutes

Cooking time: 0 minutes

Servings: 6

Ingredients:
- 1 mango, chopped
- 4 cups lettuce, chopped
- 8 oz. smoked turkey, chopped
- 2 tablespoons low-fat yogurt
- 1 teaspoon smoked paprika

Directions:
1. Mix up all ingredients in the bowls and transfer them in the serving plates.

Nutrition: 88 calories, 7.1g protein, 11.2g carbohydrates, 1.9g fat, 1.3g fiber, 25mg cholesterol, 350mg sodium, 262mg potassium.

Avocado Salad

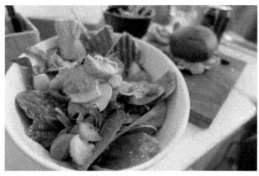

Preparation time: 5 minutes

Cooking time: 0 minutes

Servings: 4

Ingredients:

- 1/2 teaspoon ground black pepper
- 1 avocado, peeled, pitted and sliced
- 4 cups lettuce, chopped
- 1 cup black olives, pitted and halved
- 1 cup tomatoes, chopped
- 1 tablespoon olive oil

Directions:

1. Put all ingredients in the salad bowl and mix up well.

Nutrition: 197 calories,1.9g protein, 10g carbohydrates, 17.1g fat, 5.4g fiber, 0mg cholesterol, 301mg sodium, 434mg potassium.

Berry Salad With Shrimps

Preparation time: 7 minutes

Cooking time: 0 minutes

Servings: 4

Ingredients:

- 1 cup corn kernels, cooked
- 1 endive, shredded
- 1 pound shrimp, cooked
- 1 tablespoon lime juice

- 2 cups raspberries, halved
- 2 tablespoons olive oil
- 1 tablespoon parsley, chopped

Directions:

1. Put all ingredients from the list above in the salad bowl and shake well.

Nutrition: 283 calories,29.5g protein, 21.2g carbohydrates, 10.1g fat, 9.1g fiber, 239mg cholesterol, 313mg sodium, 803mg potassium.

Sliced Mushrooms Salad

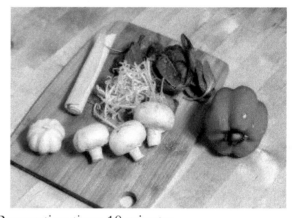

Preparation time: 10 minutes

Cooking time: 20 minutes

Servings: 4

Ingredients:

- 1 cup mushrooms, sliced
- 1 tablespoon margarine
- 1 cup lettuce, chopped
- 1 teaspoon lemon juice
- 1 tablespoon fresh dill, chopped
- 1 teaspoon cumin seeds

Directions:

1. Melt the margarine in the skillet.
2. Add mushrooms and lemon juice. Sauté the vegetables for 20 minutes over the medium heat.
3. Then transfer the cooked mushrooms to the salad bowl, add lettuce, dill, and cumin seeds.

4. Stir the salad well.

Nutrition: 35 calories,0.9g protein, 1.7g carbohydrates, 3.1g fat, 0.5g fiber, 0mg cholesterol, 38mg sodium, 113mg potassium.

Tender Green Beans Salad

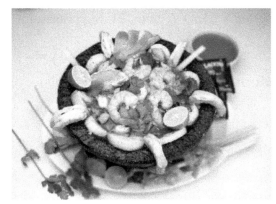

Preparation time: 5 minutes

Cooking time: 0 minutes

Servings: 8

Ingredients:

- 2 cups green beans, trimmed, chopped, cooked
- 2 tablespoons olive oil
- 2 pounds shrimp, cooked, peeled
- 1 cup tomato, chopped
- 1/4 cup apple cider vinegar

Directions:

1. Mix up all ingredients together.
2. Then transfer the salad in the salad bowl.

Nutrition: 179 calories,26.5g protein, 4.6g carbohydrates, 5.5g fat, 1.2g fiber, 239mg cholesterol, 280mg sodium, 308mg potassium.

Spinach And Chicken Salad

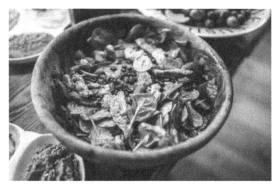

Preparation time: 7 minutes

Cooking time: 0 minutes

Servings: 4

Ingredients:

- 1 tablespoon olive oil
- A pinch of black pepper
- 1-pound chicken breast, cooked, skinless, boneless, shredded
- 1 pound cherry tomatoes, halved
- 1 red onion, sliced
- 3 cups spinach, chopped
- 1 tablespoon lemon juice
- 1 tablespoon nuts, chopped

Directions:

1. Put all ingredients in the salad bowl and gently stir with the help of a spatula.

Nutrition: 209 calories, 26.4g protein, 8.4g carbohydrates, 7.8g fat, 2.7g fiber, 73mg cholesterol, 97mg sodium, 872mg potassium.

Cilantro Salad

Preparation time: 10 minutes

Cooking time: 8 minutes

Servings: 4

Ingredients:

- 1 tablespoon avocado oil

- 1 pound shrimp, peeled and deveined
- 2 cups lettuce, chopped
- 1 tablespoon balsamic vinegar
- 1 tablespoon lemon juice
- 1 cup fresh cilantro, chopped

Directions:

1. Heat up a pan with the oil over medium heat, add the shrimps and cook them for 4 minutes per side or until they are light brown.

2. Transfer the shrimps to the salad bowl and add all remaining ingredients from the list above. Shake the salad.

Nutrition: 146 calories,26.1g protein, 3g carbohydrates, 2.5g fat, 0.5g fiber, 239mg cholesterol, 281mg sodium, 270mg potassium.

Iceberg Salad

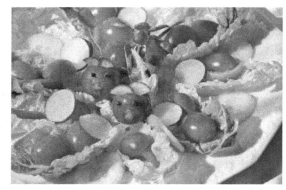

Preparation time: 10 minutes

Cooking time: 0 minutes

Servings: 4

Ingredients:
- 1 cup iceberg lettuce, chopped
- 2 oz. scallions, chopped
- 1 cup carrot, shredded
- 1 cup radish, sliced
- 2 tablespoons red vinegar
- 1/4 cup olive oil

Directions:

1. Make the dressing: mix up olive oil and red vinegar.
2. Then mix up all remaining ingredients in the salad bowl.
3. Sprinkle the salad with dressing.

Nutrition: 130 calories,0.8g protein, 5.1g carbohydrates, 12.7g fat, 1.6g fiber, 0mg cholesterol, 33mg sodium, 214mg potassium.

Seafood Salad With Grapes

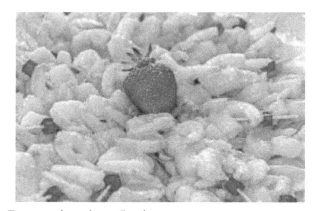

Preparation time: 5 minutes

Cooking time: 0 minutes

Servings: 4

Ingredients:
- 2 tablespoons low-fat mayonnaise
- 2 teaspoons chili powder
- 1-pound shrimp, cooked, peeled
- 1 cup green grapes, halved
- 1 oz. nuts, chopped

Directions:

1. Mix up all ingredients in the mixing bowl and transfer the salad to the serving plates.

Nutrition: 225 calories,27.4g protein, 9.9g carbohydrates, 8.3g fat, 1.3g fiber, 241mg cholesterol, 390mg sodium, 304mg potassium.

Fennel Bulb Salad

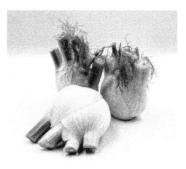

Preparation time: 10 minutes

Cooking time: 0 minutes

Servings: 4

Ingredients: 2 fennel bulbs, chopped
- 1 cup fresh parsley, chopped
- 1 tablespoon olive oil
- 1/2 cups walnuts, chopped
- 1 oz. low-fat feta cheese, crumbled

Directions:

1. Put all ingredients in the salad bowl. Mix up the mixture.

Nutrition: 181 calories,6.9g protein, 11.3g carbohydrates, 13.8g fat, 5.2g fiber, 3mg cholesterol, 156mg sodium, 649mg potassium.

Russet Potato Salad

Preparation time: 10 minutes

Cooking time: 20 minutes

Servings: 4

Ingredients:
- 2 tomatoes, chopped
- 2 cups spinach, chopped
- 2 scallions, chopped
- 3 russet potatoes
- 1 tablespoon olive oil
- 1 tablespoon apple cider vinegar

Directions:

1. Bake the potatoes in the preheated to 400F oven for 20 minutes. Meanwhile, mix up all remaining ingredients in the salad bowl.
2. Cool the potatoes, peel them, and cut into cubes. Add to the salad and mix up well.

Nutrition: 158 calories,3.8g protein, 28.6g carbohydrates, 3.9g fat, 5.1g fiber, 0mg cholesterol, 26mg sodium, 903mg potassium.

Sweet Persimmon Salad

Preparation time: 10 minutes

Cooking time: 0 minutes

Servings: 4

Ingredients:
- 1/3 cup pomegranate seeds
- 2 persimmons, chopped
- 5 cups baby arugula
- 4 navel oranges, peeled and cut into segments
- 3 tablespoons pine nuts
- 2 tablespoons orange juice
- 1/4 teaspoon ground cinnamon
- 1 tablespoon liquid honey

Directions:

1. Put all ingredients in the big salad bowl and mix it up.

Nutrition: 180 calories,3.5g protein, 34.8g carbohydrates, 4.9g fat, 5.2g fiber, 0mg cholesterol, 7mg sodium, 521mg potassium.

Mint Seafood Salad

Preparation time: 5 minutes

Cooking time: 18 minutes

Servings: 4

Ingredients: 1 cup of water

- 2 tablespoons olive oil
- 2 cups broccoli florets
- 1 cup shrimps, peeled
- 4 cherry tomatoes, halved
- 1/2 cup Kalamata olives, chopped
- 1 tablespoon mint, chopped

Directions:

1. Bring the water to boil, add broccoli, and cook it for 10 minutes.
2. Then add shrimps and cook the ingredients for 5 minutes more.
3. Drain the water and transfer the broccoli and shrimps to the salad bowl.
4. Add all remaining ingredients and shake the salad.

Nutrition: 118 calories,2.6g protein, 9g carbohydrates, 9.2g fat, 3.3g fiber, 0mg cholesterol, 170mg sodium, 444mg potassium.

Green Dill Salad

Preparation time: 10 minutes

Cooking time: 4 minutes

Servings: 4

Ingredients:

- 1/2 cup dill, chopped
- 1 cup asparagus, chopped
- 1 tablespoon olive oil
- 1 tablespoon lemon juice
- 1 tablespoon canola oil
- 1 teaspoon sesame seeds
- 1 cup lettuce, chopped

Directions:

1. Roast the asparagus with olive oil in the skillet for 4 minutes and transfer it in the salad bowl.
2. Add all remaining ingredients and stir the salad well.

Nutrition: 90 calories,2.2g protein, 5.3g carbohydrates, 7.7g fat, 1.7g fiber, 0mg cholesterol, 15mg sodium, 294mg potassium.

Fish And Mushrooms Salad

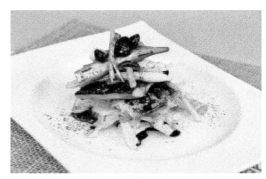

Preparation time: 10 minutes

Cooking time: 20 minutes

Servings: 4

Ingredients:

- 2 salmon fillets, chopped
- 1 tablespoon olive oil
- 1/2 teaspoon oregano, dried
- 8 ounces white mushrooms, sliced
- 1 tablespoon lemon juice
- 1 cup black olives, pitted and halved
- 1 tablespoon parsley, chopped
- 1/2 cup of water

Directions:

1. Put salmon and mushrooms in the baking pan.
2. Add water and oregano. Bake the ingredients for 20 minutes at 365F.
3. Then transfer the cooked ingredients to the salad bowl.
4. Add all remaining ingredients and mix up.

Nutrition: 211 calories, 20g protein, 2.4g carbohydrates, 13.4g fat, 1.2g fiber, 55mg cholesterol, 339mg sodium, 500mg potassium.

CHAPTER 10:

Poultry

Chili Turkey Fillet

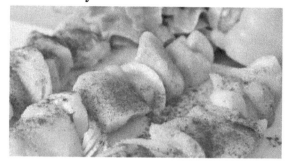

Preparation time: 5 minutes

Cooking time: 40 minutes

Servings: 4

Ingredients:

- 12 oz. turkey fillet, chopped
- 1 cup low-fat milk
- 2 cups asparagus, chopped
- 1 teaspoon chili powder
- 2 tablespoons olive oil
- 1/2 teaspoon cayenne pepper

Directions:

1. Heat up a pan with the oil over medium-high heat, add the turkey and cayenne pepper, toss and cook for 5 minutes.
2. Add all remaining ingredients and cook the meal over the medium heat for 35 minutes.

Nutrition: 182 calories,21.3g protein, 6.1g carbohydrates, 8.2g fat, 1.7g fiber, 47mg cholesterol, 227mg sodium, 244mg potassium.

Chicken Topped With Coconut

Preparation time: 10 minutes

Cooking time: 50 minutes

Servings: 8

Ingredients:

- 3 tablespoons olive oil
- 8 chicken thighs, skinless, boneless
- 1/2 teaspoon ground black pepper
- 1 teaspoon garlic powder
- 1 cup low-fat yogurt
- 1 tablespoon coconut shred

Directions:

1. Heat up olive oil in the saucepan.
2. Add chicken thighs and sprinkle them with ground black pepper and garlic powder.
3. Cook the chicken for 5 minutes per side.
4. Add yogurt and coconut shred. Close the lid and simmer the meal for 40 minutes over the low heat.

Nutrition: 350 calories,44.1g protein, 3.2g carbohydrates, 16.6g fat, 0.1g fiber, 132mg cholesterol, 175mg sodium, 432mg potassium.

Chicken With Red Onion

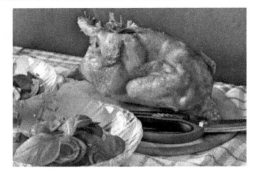

Preparation time: 10 minutes

Cooking time: 30 minutes

Servings: 4

Ingredients:

- 1-pound chicken breasts, skinless, boneless, roughly cubed
- 3 red onions, sliced
- 2 tablespoons olive oil
- 1 cup of water
- 1 teaspoon dried thyme

Directions:

1. Heat up a pan with the oil over medium heat, add the onions and sauté for 10 minutes stirring often.
2. Add the chicken and cook for 3 minutes more.
3. Then add water, thyme, and stir the meal well.
4. Cook it for 15 minutes more.

Nutrition: 223 calories, 25g protein, 7.9g carbohydrates, 9.9g fat, 1.9g fiber, 73mg cholesterol, 63mg sodium, 543mg potassium.

Clove Chicken

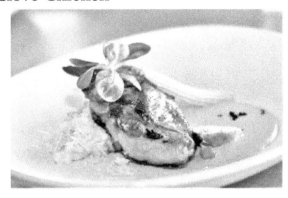

Preparation time: 10 minutes

Cooking time: 25 minutes

Servings: 4

Ingredients:

- 1-pound chicken fillet, sliced
- 1 teaspoon ground clove
- 1 tablespoon avocado oil
- 1/2 cup tomato, chopped
- 1/4 cup of water

Directions:

1. Heat up oil in the saucepan.
2. Add chicken and ground clove and stir the meal for 10 minutes.
3. After this, add tomato and water.
4. Close the lid and simmer the meal for 15 minutes more.

Nutrition: 226 calories, 33.1g protein, 1.4g carbohydrates, 9g fat, 0.6g fiber, 101mg cholesterol, 100mg sodium, 346mg potassium.

Rice With Turkey

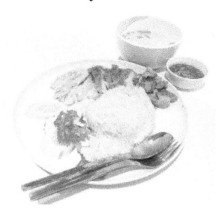

Preparation time: 10 minutes

Cooking time: 25 minutes

Ingredients:

- 1-pound turkey fillet, chopped
- 1 cup wild rice
- 2 cup of water
- 1 teaspoon chili powder
- 2 garlic cloves, minced
- 2 tablespoons olive oil
- 1 tablespoon low-fat yogurt

Directions:

1. Heat up a pan with the oil over medium heat, add turkey and chili powder.
2. Cook the ingredients for 5 minutes.
3. After this, add all remaining ingredients, stir well, and close the lid.
4. Cook the meal for 40 minutes over the low heat.

Nutrition: 343 calories, 27.2g protein, 38.1g carbohydrates, 8g fat, 0.9g fiber, 59mg cholesterol, 272mg sodium, 82mg potassium.

Apple Chicken

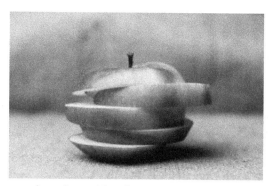

Preparation time: 10 minutes

Cooking time: 40 minutes

Ingredients:

- 4 chicken thighs, skinless, boneless
- 1/2 teaspoon ground black pepper
- 1 cup apples, chopped
- 1/2 cup apple juice
- 1 teaspoon margarine

Directions:

1. Heat up margarine in the saucepan.
2. Add chicken and roast it for 5 minutes per side.
3. After this, add all remaining ingredients and close the lid.
4. Simmer the chicken for 30 minutes.

Nutrition: 330 calories, 42.5g protein, 11.4g carbohydrates, 11.9g fat, 1.5g fiber, 130mg cholesterol, 139mg sodium, 449mg potassium.

Turkey And Savoy Cabbage Mix

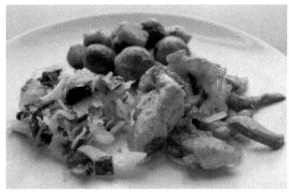

Preparation time: 10 minutes

Cooking time: 30 minutes

Servings: 4

Ingredients:

- 10 oz. turkey fillet, sliced
- 1 cup of water
- 1 tablespoon olive oil
- 1 cup Savoy cabbage, shredded
- 1 teaspoon chili powder
- 1 tablespoon margarine

Directions:

1. Put all ingredients in the baking pan and cover with the foil.
2. Bake the meal for 30 minutes at 385F.

Nutrition: 129 calories, 15g protein, 1.4g carbohydrates, 6.8g fat, 0.7g fiber, 37mg cholesterol, 205mg sodium, 44mg potassium.

Soft Sage Turkey

Preparation time: 10 minutes

Cooking time: 35 minutes

Servings: 4

Ingredients:

- 1-pound turkey fillet, chopped
- 1 tablespoon margarine, melted

- 1 teaspoon dried sage
- 1 tablespoon olive oil

Directions:

1. Mix up olive oil, margarine, and sage in the shallow bowl.
2. Mix up turkey fillet and oil mixture together, and transfer in the baking pan.
3. Bake the meal at 375F for 35 minutes.

Nutrition: 163 calories,23.6g protein, 0.1g carbohydrates, 6.9g fat, 0.1g fiber, 59mg cholesterol, 290mg sodium, 3mg potassium.

Thai Style Chicken Cubes

Preparation time: 10 minutes

Cooking time: 35 minutes

Servings: 6

Ingredients:

- 16 oz. chicken fillet, cubed
- 1 tablespoon scallions, chopped
- 1/2 cup Thai chili sauce

Directions:

1. Heat up a pan over medium-high heat, add chicken and roast it for 5 minutes on each side, transfer to a baking dish, add chili sauce and scallions, toss well and transfer the meal to the preheated to 390F oven.

2. Bake the meal for 35 minutes.

Nutrition: 145 calories, 21.9g protein, 0.3g carbohydrates, 5.6g fat, 0g fiber, 67mg cholesterol, 70mg sodium, 186mg potassium.

Ginger Sauce Chicken

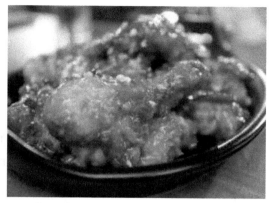

Preparation time: 10 minutes

Cooking time: 35 minutes

Servings: 4

Ingredients:

- 1 pound chicken breast, skinless, boneless, chopped
- 1 tablespoon ginger, grated
- 1 tablespoon olive oil
- 1 teaspoon minced garlic
- 1 teaspoon smoked paprika
- 1/4 cup low-fat yogurt

Directions:

1. Heat up olive oil in the skillet. Add chicken and cook it for 5 minutes per side.
2. Then add ginger, minced garlic, and smoked paprika.
3. Stir the chicken well and add yogurt.
4. Close the lid and cook the meal for 25 minutes.

Nutrition: 177 calories, 25.2g protein, 2.6g carbohydrates, 6.7g fat, 0.4g fiber, 74mg cholesterol, 69mg sodium, 489mg potassium.

Quinoa Chicken

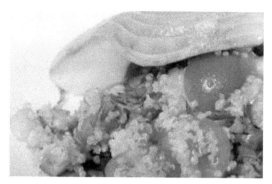

Preparation time: 10 minutes

Cooking time: 30 minutes

Servings: 6

Ingredients:

- 1-pound chicken breast, skinless, boneless, chopped
- 1 tablespoon avocado oil
- 1 cup quinoa
- 2 cups of water
- 1 tablespoon lemon juice
- 1 tablespoon dill, chopped
- 1/2 teaspoon ground black pepper
- 1 tablespoon red curry paste

Directions:

1. Heat up a pan with the oil over medium-high heat, add the chicken and brown it for 10 minutes.
2. Add all remaining ingredients and stir the mixture until homogenous.
3. Close the lid and simmer the chicken for 20 minutes over the medium-high heat.

Nutrition: 206 calories, 20.2g protein, 19.3g carbohydrates, 4.7g fat, 2.2g fiber, 48mg cholesterol, 174mg sodium, 470mg potassium.

Parsnip Turkey

Preparation time: 10 minutes

Cooking time: 25 minutes

Servings: 4

Ingredients:

- 12 oz. turkey fillet, sliced
- 2 parsnips, chopped
- 1 tablespoon parsley, chopped
- 2 tablespoons sesame oil
- 1 onion, chopped
- 1 cup of water

Directions:

1. Heat up the pan with the oil over medium heat, add the onion and sauté for 5 minutes.

2. Add the turkey, toss and cook for 5 minutes more.

3. Add all remaining ingredients, close the lid and simmer the meal for 15 minutes.

Nutrition: 177 calories, 18.4g protein, 8.6g carbohydrates, 7.3g fat, 2.3g fiber, 44mg cholesterol, 199mg sodium, 171mg potassium.

Chopped Chicken

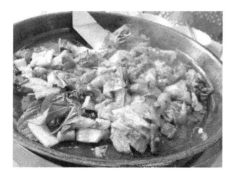

Preparation time: 10 minutes

Cooking time: 25 minutes

Servings: 4

Ingredients:

- 1 teaspoon ground paprika
- 1 teaspoon tomato paste
- 1 tablespoon olive oil
- 1-pound chicken fillet, chopped

Directions:

1. Mix up all ingredients in the baking pan and cover with foil.
2. Bake the chopped chicken for 30 minutes at 375F.

Nutrition: 248 calories, 33g protein, 0.6g carbohydrates, 12g fat, 0.3g fiber, 101mg cholesterol, 99mg sodium, 301mg potassium.

Chicken In Bell Pepper

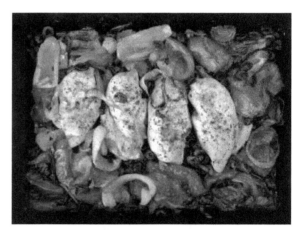

Preparation time: 10 minutes

Cooking time: 35 minutes

Servings: 5

Ingredients:

- 16 oz. chicken breast, skinless, boneless, chopped
- 2 cups bell pepper, chopped
- 1 teaspoon dried thyme
- 1 teaspoon smoked paprika
- 1 teaspoon ground black pepper
- 1 teaspoon dried oregano
- 1 cup low-fat yogurt

Directions:

1. Mix up all ingredients in the baking pan and flatten well.
2. Bake the chicken for 35 minutes at 375F.

Nutrition: 157 calories, 22.7g protein, 7.9g carbohydrates, 3.1g fat, 1.1g fiber, 61mg cholesterol, 82mg sodium, 562mg potassium.

Chickpea Chicken

Preparation time: 10 minutes

Cooking time: 25 minutes

Servings: 4

Ingredients:

- 1 cup chickpeas, cooked

- 1/2 cup of water

- 1-pound chicken breast, skinless, boneless, chopped

- 1 teaspoon ground black pepper

- 1 teaspoon oregano, dried

- 1 teaspoon nutmeg, ground

- 1 tablespoon margarine

Directions:

1. Heat up margarine in the saucepan and add chicken breast, ground black pepper, oregano, and nutmeg.
2. Roast the chicken for 10 minutes.
3. Then stir well, and add water and chickpeas.
4. Close the lid and cook the meal for 15 minutes more.

Nutrition: 342 calories, 33.9g protein, 31.2g carbohydrates, 9g fat, 9.1g fiber, 73mg cholesterol, 105mg sodium, 874mg potassium.

Carrot Chicken

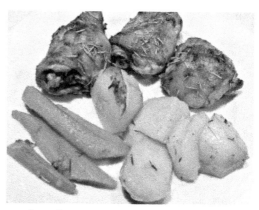

Preparation time: 10 minutes

Cooking time: 60 minutes

Servings: 8

Ingredients:

- 2 onions, chopped
- 8 chicken thighs, skinless, boneless
- 1 teaspoon minced garlic
- 1 tablespoon margarine
- 1/2 teaspoon chili flakes
- 1 cup of water
- 1 cup carrot, shredded

Directions:

1. Melt margarine in the saucepan and add the onion. Cook it for 5 minutes.
2. Then add all remaining ingredients and stir the mixture well.
3. Cook it with the closed lid for 55 minutes over the low heat.

Nutrition: 307 calories, 42.7g protein, 4.1g carbohydrates, 12.3g fat, 0.9g fiber, 130mg cholesterol, 154mg sodium, 442mg potassium.

Turkey With Olive

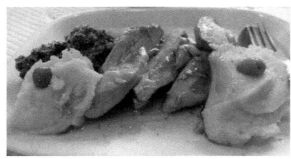

Preparation time: 10 minutes

Cooking time: 35 minutes

Servings: 4

Ingredients:

- 1 cup green olives, pitted and halved

- 1 pound turkey fillet, sliced

- 1 tablespoon parsley, chopped

- 1 cup tomato puree

- 1 tablespoon olive oil

Directions:

1. Grease a baking dish with the oil.

2. Add all remaining ingredients in the baking pan, flatten well, and cover with foil.

3. Bake the meal ta 385F for 35 minutes.

Nutrition: 200 calories, 24.9g protein, 7.8g carbohydrates, 7.8g fat, 2.3g fiber, 59mg cholesterol, 568mg sodium, 282mg potassium.

CHAPTER 11:

Beef, Pork and Lamb

Authentic Pepper Steak

Preparation time: 5 Minutes

Cooking Time: 30 minutes

Servings: 4

Ingredients:

- 1 tbsp. sesame oil
- 80 oz. sliced mushroom
- 1 c. water
- 1 sliced red pepper piece
- 1 pack onion soup mix
- 1 lb. de-boned beef eye of round steak
- 1 tbsp. minced garlic

Directions:

1. Add the listed ingredients to your Instant Pot
2. Lock up the lid and cook on HIGH pressure for 20 minutes
3. Release the pressure naturally over 10 minutes
4. Serve the pepper steak and enjoy!

Nutrition:

Calories: 222, Fat:15 g, Carbs:5 g, Protein:36 g, Sugars:1.56 g, Sodium:556 mg

Lamb Chops With Rosemary

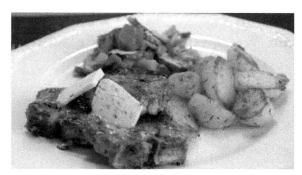

Preparation time: 5 Minutes

Cooking Time: 15 minutes

Servings: 4

Ingredients:

- 1 lb. lamb chops
- 1/2 tsp. freshly ground black pepper
- 1 tbsp. olive oil
- 5 garlic cloves
- 1 tbsp. chopped fresh rosemary

Directions:

1. Adjust oven rack to the top third of the oven. Preheat broiler. Line a baking sheet with foil.
2. Place the garlic, rosemary, pepper, and olive oil into a small bowl and stir well to combine.
3. Place the lamb chops on a baking sheet and brush half of the garlic-rosemary mixture equally between the chops, coating well. Place the sheet beneath broiler and broil 4–5 minutes.
4. Remove from oven and carefully flip over the chops. Divide the remaining

garlic-rosemary mixture evenly between the chops and spread to coat. Return pan to oven and broil for another 3 minutes.

5. Remove from oven and serve immediately.

Nutrition:

Calories: 185, Fat: 9 g, Carbs:1 g, Protein: 23 g, Sugars: 0 g, Sodium:72.8 mg

Cane Wrapped Around In Prosciutto

Preparation time: 3 Minutes

Cooking Time: 5 minutes

Servings: 4

Ingredients:

- 80 oz. sliced prosciutto
- 1 lb. thick asparagus

Directions:

1. The first step here is to prepare your instant pot by pouring in about 2 cups of water
2. Take the asparagus and wrap them up in prosciutto spears. Once all of the asparagus are wrapped, gently place the processed asparaguses in the cooking basket inside your pot in layers. Turn up the heat to a high temperature and when there is a pressure build up, take down the heat and let it cook for about 2-3 minutes at the high pressure. Once the timer runs out, gently open the cover of the pressure cooker
3. Take out the steamer basket from the pot instantly and toss the asparaguses on a plate to serve
4. Eat warm or let them come down to room temperature

Nutrition:

Calories: 212, Fat:14 g, Carbs:11 g, Protein:12 g, Sugars: 367.6 g, Sodium: 0 mg

Beef Veggie Pot Meal

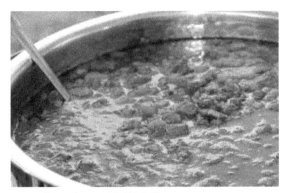

Preparation time: 45-50 Minutes

Cooking Time: 40 minutes

Servings:2-3

Ingredients:

- 1 tsp. butter
- 1/4 shredded cabbage head
- 2 peeled and sliced carrots
- 1 tbsp. flour
- 4 tbsps. sour cream
- 1 chopped onion
- 10 oz. sliced and boiled beef tenderloin

Directions:

1. In a saucepan; add the butter, cabbage, carrots, and onions.
2. Cook on medium-high heat until the veggies get softened.
3. Add the beef meat and stir the mix.
4. In a mixing bowl, beat the cream with flour until smooth.
5. Add the sauce over the beef.
6. Cover and cook for 40 minutes.
7. Serve warm.

Nutrition:

Calories: 245.5, Fat:10.2 g, Carbs:18.4 g, Protein:19.0 g, Sugars:5.5 g, Sodium:188.2 mg

Braised Beef Shanks

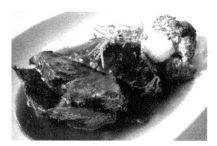

Preparation time: 10 Minutes

Cooking Time: 4-6 hours

Servings: 2

Ingredients:

- Freshly ground black pepper
- 5 minced garlic cloves
- 1 1/2 lbs. lean beef shanks
- 2 sprigs fresh rosemary
- 1 c. low-fat, low-sodium beef broth
- 1 tbsp. fresh lime juice

Directions:

1. In a slow cooker, add all ingredients and mix. Set the slow cooker on low.
2. Cover and cook for 4-6 hours.

Nutrition: Calories: 50, Fat:1 g, Carbs: 0.8 g, Protein:8 g, Sugars: 0 g, Sodium:108 mg

Beef With Mushrooms

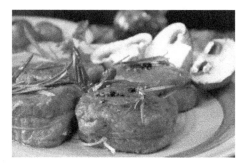

Preparation time: 15 Minutes

Cooking Time: 8 hours

Servings: 8

Ingredients:

- 2 c. salt-free tomato paste
- 2 c. sliced fresh mushrooms
- 2 c. low-fat, low-sodium beef broth
- 2 lbs. cubed lean beef stew meat
- 1 c. chopped fresh parsley leaves
- Freshly ground black pepper
- 4 minced garlic cloves

Directions:

1. In a slow cooker add all ingredients except lemon juice and, stir to combine.
2. Set the slow cooker on low.
3. Cover and cook for about 8 hours.
4. Serve hot with the drizzling of lemon juice

Nutrition:

Calories: 260, Fat:12 g, Carbs:18 g, Protein:44 g, Sugars:4 g, Sodium:480 mg

Lemony Braised Beef Roast

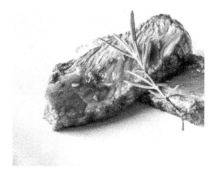

Preparation time: 15 Minutes

Cooking Time: 6-8 hours

Servings: 6

Ingredients:

- 1 tbsp. minced fresh rosemary
- 1/2 c. low-fat, low-sodium beef broth
- Freshly ground black pepper

- 2 lbs. lean beef pot roast
- 1 sliced onion
- 2 minced garlic cloves
- 1/4 c. fresh lemon juice
- 1 tsp. ground cumin

Directions:

1. In a large slow cooker, add all ingredients and mix well.
2. Set the slow cooker on low.
3. Cover and cook for about 6-8 hours.

Nutrition:

Calories: 344, Fat: 2.8 g, Carbs:18 g, Protein: 32 g, Sugars: 2.4 g, Sodium: 278 mg

Grilled Fennel-Cumin Lamb Chops

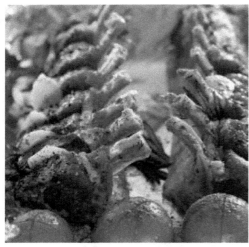

Preparation time: 10 Minutes

Cooking Time: 30 minutes

Servings: 2

Ingredients:

- 1/4 tsp. salt
- 1 minced large garlic clove
- 1/8 tsp. cracked black pepper
- ¾ tsp. crushed fennel seeds
- 1/4 tsp. ground coriander
- 4-6 sliced lamb rib chops
- ¾ tsp. ground cumin

Directions:

1. Trim fat from chops. Place the chops on a plate.
2. In a small bowl combine the garlic, fennel seeds, cumin, salt, coriander, and black pepper. Sprinkle the mixture evenly over chops; rub in with your fingers. Cover the chops with plastic wrap and marinate in the refrigerator at least 30 minutes or up to 24 hours.
3. Grill chops on the rack of an uncovered grill directly over medium coals until chops are desired doneness.

Nutrition:

Calories: 239, Fat:12 g, Carbs: 2 g, Protein: 29 g, Sugars: 0 g, Sodium:409 mg

Beef Heart

Preparation time: 40 Minutes

Cooking Time: 30 minutes

Servings: 4

Ingredients:

- 1 chopped large onion
- 1 c. water
- 2 peeled and chopped tomatoes
- 1 boiled beef heart
- 2 tbsps. tomato paste

Directions:

1. Boil the beef heart until half-done.
2. Sauté the onions with tomatoes until soft.
3. Cut the beef heart into cubes and add to tomato and onion mixture. Add water and tomato paste. Stew on low heat for 30 minutes.

Nutrition:

Calories: 138, Fat:3 g, Carbs:0.1 g, Protein:24.2 g, Sugars: 0 g, Sodium:50.2 mg

Jerk Beef And Plantain Kabobs

Preparation time: 10 Minutes

Cooking Time: 15 minutes

Servings: 4

Ingredients:

- 2 peeled and sliced ripe plantains
- 2 tbsps. Red wine vinegar
- Lime wedges
- 1 tbsp. cooking oil
- 1 sliced medium red onion
- 12 oz. sliced boneless beef sirloin steak
- 1 tbsp. Jamaican jerk seasoning

Directions:

1. Trim fat from meat. Cut into 1-inch pieces. In a small bowl, stir together red wine vinegar, oil, and jerk seasoning. Toss meat cubes with half of the vinegar mixture. On long skewers, alternately thread meat, plantain chunks, and onion wedges, leaving a 1/4-inch space between pieces.
2. Brush plantains and onion wedges with remaining vinegar mixture.
3. Place skewers on the rack of an uncovered grill directly over medium coals. Grill for 12 to 15 minutes or until meat is desired doneness, turning occasionally.
4. Serve with lime wedges.

Nutrition:

Calories: 260, Fat: 7 g, Carbs: 21 g, Protein:26 g, Sugars: 2.5 g, Sodium: 358 mg

Beef Pot

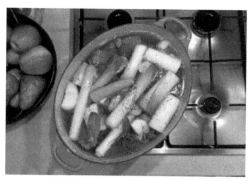

Preparation time: 10 Minutes

Cooking Time: 40 minutes

Servings: 2

Ingredients:

- 4 tbsps. Sour cream
- 1/4 shredded cabbage head
- 1 tsp. butter
- 2 peeled and sliced carrots
- 1 chopped onion
- 10 oz. boiled and sliced beef tenderloin
- 1 tbsp. flour

Directions:

1. Sauté the cabbage, carrots and onions in butter.
2. Spray a pot with cooking spray.
3. In layers place the sautéed vegetables, then beef, then another layer of vegetables.
4. Beat the sour cream with flour until smooth and pour over the beef.
5. Cover and bake at 400F for 40 minutes.

Nutrition:

Calories: 210, Fat: 30 g, Carbs:4 g, Protein:14 g, Sugars:1 g, Sodium: 600 mg

Beef With Cucumber Raita

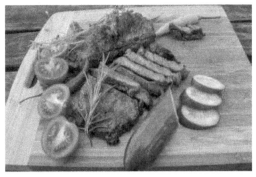

Preparation time: 10 Minutes

Cooking Time: 30 minutes

Servings: 2

Ingredients:

- 1/2 tsp. lemon-pepper seasoning
- 1/4 c. coarsely shredded unpeeled cucumber
- Black pepper and salt
- 1 tbsp. finely chopped red onion
- 1/4 tsp. sugar
- 1 lb. sliced de-boned beef sirloin steak
- 8 oz. plain fat-free yogurt
- 1 tbsp. snipped fresh mint

Directions:

1. Preheat broiler.
2. In a small bowl combine yogurt, cucumber, onion, snipped mint, and sugar. Season to taste with salt and pepper; set aside
3. Trim fat from meat. Sprinkle meat with lemon-pepper seasoning.
4. Place meat on the unheated rack of a broiler pan. Broil 3 to 4 inches from heat, turning meat over after half of the broiling time.
5. Allow 15 to 17 minutes for medium-rare (145 degree F) and 20 to 22 minutes for medium (160 degree F).
6. Cut steak across the grain into thin slices.
7. Serve and enjoy.

Nutrition:

Calories: 176, Fat:3 g, Carbs:5 g, Protein:28 g, Sugars: 8.9 g, Sodium: 88.3 mg

Bistro Beef Tenderloin

Preparation time: 10 Minutes

Cooking Time: 45 minutes

Servings: 12

Ingredients:

- 2 tbsps. Extra-virgin olive oil
- 2 tbsps. Dijon mustard
- 1 tsp. kosher salt
- 2/3 c. chopped mixed fresh herbs
- 3 lbs. trimmed beef tenderloin
- 1/2 tsp. freshly ground pepper

Directions:

1. Preheat oven to 400F.
2. Tie kitchen string around tenderloin in three places so it doesn't flatten while roasting.
3. Rub the tenderloin with oil; pat on salt and pepper. Place in a large roasting pan.
4. Roast until a thermometer inserted into the thickest part of the tenderloin registers 140F for medium-rare, about 45 minutes, turning two or three times during roasting to ensure even cooking.
5. Transfer to a cutting board; let rest for 10 minutes. Remove the string.
6. Place herbs on a large plate. Coat the tenderloin evenly with mustard; then roll in the herbs, pressing gently to adhere. Slice and serve.

Nutrition:

Calories: 280, Fat: 20.6 g, Carbs: 0.9 g, Protein: 22.2 g, Sugars: 0 g, Sodium:160 mg

The Surprising No "Noodle" Lasagna

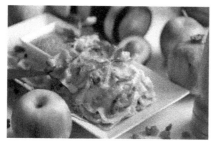

Preparation time: 10 Minutes

Cooking Time: 10 minutes

Servings: 8

Ingredients:

- 1/2 c. Parmesan cheese
- 2 minced garlic cloves
- 8 oz. sliced mozzarella
- 1 lb. ground beef
- 25 oz. marinara sauce
- 1 small sized onion
- 1 1/2 c. ricotta cheese
- 1 large sized egg

Directions:

1. Set your pot to Sauté mode and add garlic, onion and ground beef
2. Take a small bowl and add ricotta and parmesan with egg and mix
3. Drain the grease and transfer the beef to a 1 and a 1/2 quart soufflé dish
4. Add marinara sauce to the browned meat and reserve half
5. Top the remaining meat sauce with half of your mozzarella cheese
6. Spread half of the ricotta cheese over the mozzarella layer
7. Top with the remaining meat sauce
8. Add a final layer of mozzarella cheese on top
9. Spread any remaining ricotta cheese mix over the mozzarella
10. Carefully add this mixture to your Soufflé Dish
11. Pour 1 cup of water to your pot
12. Place it over a trivet
13. Lock up the lid and cook on HIGH pressure for 10 minutes
14. Release the pressure naturally over 10 minutes
15. Serve and enjoy!

Nutrition:

Calories: 607, Fat: 23 g, Carbs: 65 g, Protein:33 g, Sugars: 0.31 g, Sodium:128 mg

Lamb Chops With Kale

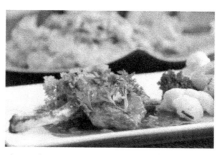

Preparation time: 10 Minutes

Cooking Time: 35 minutes

Servings: 4

Ingredients:

- 1 tbsp. olive oil
- 1 sliced yellow onion
- 1 c. torn kale
- 2 tbsps. low-sodium tomato paste
- 1/4 tsp. black pepper
- 1/2 c. low-sodium veggie stock
- 1 lb. lamb chops

Directions:

1. Grease a roasting pan with the oil, arrange the lamb chops inside, also add the kale and the other ingredients and toss gently.
2. Bake everything at 390F for 35 minutes, divide between plates and serve.

Nutrition:

Calories: 275, Fat:11.8 g, Carbs:7.3 g, Protein:33.6 g, Sugars:0.1 g, Sodium:280 mg

Beef & Vegetable Stir-Fry

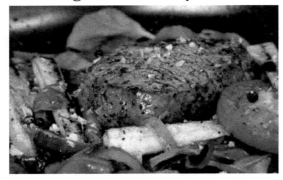

Preparation time: 20 Minutes

Cooking Time: 30 minutes

Servings: 4

Ingredients:

- 1 lb. thinly sliced skirt steak
- 2 tbsps. sesame seeds
- ¾ c. stir-fry sauce
- 1 thinly sliced red bell pepper
- 2 thinly sliced scallions
- 2 tbsps. canola oil
- 1/4 tsp. ground black pepper
- 1 sliced broccoli head
- 11/2 c. fluffy brown rice

Directions:

1. Prepare the Stir-Fry Sauce.
2. Heat the canola oil in a large wok or skillet over medium-high heat. Season the steak with the black pepper and cook for 4 minutes, until crispy on the outside and pink on the inside. Remove the steak from the skillet and place the broccoli and peppers in the hot oil. Stir-fry for 4 minutes, stirring or tossing occasionally, until crisp and slightly tender.
3. Place the steak back in the skillet with the vegetables. Pour the stir-fry sauce over the steak and vegetables and let simmer for 3 minutes. Remove from the heat.
4. Serve the stir-fry over rice and top with the scallions and sesame seeds.
5. For leftovers, divide the stir-fry evenly into microwaveable airtight containers and store in the refrigerator for up to 5 days. Reheat in the microwave on high for 2 to 3 minutes, until heated through.

Nutrition:

Calories: 408, Fat:18 g, Carbs:36 g, Protein:31 g, Sugars:5.5 g, Sodium:197 mg

Simple Veal Chops

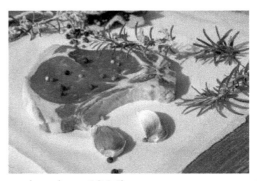

Preparation time: 10 Minutes

Cooking Time: 10 minutes

Servings: 4

Ingredients:

- 3 tbsps. essential olive oil
- Zest of 1 grated lemon
- 3 tbsps. whole-wheat flour
- 1 1/2 c. whole-wheat breadcrumbs
- Black pepper
- 1 tbsp. milk
- 4 veal rib chops
- 2 eggs

Directions:

1. Put whole-wheat flour within a bowl.
2. In another bowl, mix eggs with milk and whisk

3. In 1 / 3 bowl, mix the breadcrumbs with lemon zest.
4. Season veal chops with black pepper, dredge them in flour, and dip inside egg mix then in breadcrumbs.
5. Heat up a pan because of the oil over medium-high heat, add veal chops, cook for 2 main minutes on both sides and transfer to some baking sheet, introduce them inside oven at 350 0F, bake for quarter-hour, divide between plates and serve utilizing a side salad.
6. Enjoy!

Nutrition:

Calories: 270, Fat:6 g, Carbs:10 g, Protein:16 g, Sugars:0 g, Sodium: 320 mg

Beef And Barley Farmers Soup

Preparation time: 10 Minutes

Cooking Time: 20 minutes

Servings: 4

Ingredients:

- 1 diced onion
- 15 g sunflower oil
- 15 g balsamic vinegar
- 900 g Campbell's red and white vegetable beef soup bowl
- 2 thinly sliced green onion stalks
- 1 diced carrot
- 340 g cubed lean beef
- 1 Julienned celery stalk
- 1 Minced Garlic Clove
- 85 g pot barley

Directions:

1. Throw a cast iron pan or a deep saucepan on medium heat with the oil and cubed beef to allow the two to cook. Wait till beef is properly browned on all sides, and then add in the diced vegetables. Cover and cook

for an additional 3-5 minutes, stirring occasionally.
2. Add in a combination of the broth, vinegar, and barley; reduce flame and bring to a boil. Continue to cook for about 20 minutes, or until thickened to preferred consistency.
3. Top with chopped green onions and serve!

Nutrition:

Calories: 279, Fat:7.6 g, Carbs:28.91 g, Protein:24.82 g, Sugars:3 g, Sodium:590 mg

Simple Pork And Capers

Preparation time: 10 Minutes

Cooking Time: 10 minutes

Servings: 2

Ingredients:

- 8 oz. cubed pork
- 1 c. low-sodium chicken stock
- Black pepper
- 2 tbsps. Organic extra virgin olive oil
- 1 minced garlic oil
- 2 tbsps. Capers

Directions:

1. Heat up a pan with the oil over medium-high heat, add the pork season with black pepper and cook for 4 minutes on both sides.
2. Add garlic, capers and stock, stir and cook for 7 minutes more.
3. Divide everything between plates and serve.
4. Enjoy!

Nutrition:

Calories: 224, Fat:12 g, Carbs:12 g, Protein:10 g, Sugars:5 g, Sodium:5 mg

A "Boney" Pork Chop

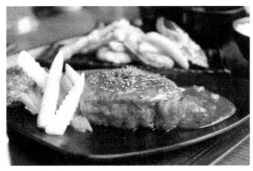

Preparation time: 20 Minutes

Cooking Time: 30 minutes

Servings: 4

Ingredients:

- 1 c. baby carrots
- Flavored vinegar
- 3 tbsps. Worcestershire sauce
- Ground pepper
- 1 chopped onion
- 4 ¾ bone-in thick pork chops
- 1/4 c. divided butter
- 1 c. vegetables

Directions:

1. Take a bowl and add pork chops, season with pepper and flavored vinegar
2. Take a skillet and place it over medium heat, add 2 teaspoon of butter and melt it
3. Toss the pork chops and brown them
4. Each side should take about 3-5 minutes
5. Set your pot to sauté mode and add 2 tablespoon of butter, add carrots and sauté them
6. Pour broth and Worcestershire
7. Add pork chops and lock up the lid
8. Cook on HIGH pressure for 13 minutes
9. Release the pressure naturally
10. Enjoy!

Nutrition:

Calories: 715, Fat:37.4 g, Carbs:2 g, Protein:20.7 g, Sugars:0 g, Sodium:276 mg

Roast And Mushrooms

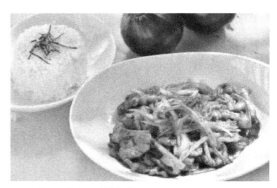

Preparation time: 10 Minutes

Cooking Time: 20 minutes

Servings: 4

Ingredients:

- 1 tsp. Italian seasoning
- 12 oz. low-sodium beef stock
- 3 1/2 lbs. pork roast
- 4 oz. sliced mushrooms

Directions:

1. In a roasting pan, combine the roast with mushrooms, stock and Italian seasoning, and toss
2. Introduce inside the oven and bake at 350F for starters hour and 20 minutes.
3. Slice the roast, divide it along while using mushroom mix between plates and serve.
4. Enjoy!

Nutrition:

Calories: 310, Fat:16 g, Carbs:10 g, Protein: 22 g, Sugars:4 g, Sodium: 600 mg

Pork And Celery Mix

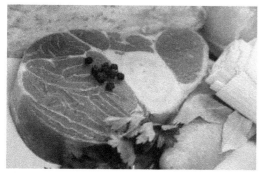

Preparation time: 10 Minutes

Cooking Time: 30 minutes

Servings: 8

Ingredients:

- 3 tsps. Fenugreek powder
- Black pepper
- 1 tbsp. organic olive oil
- 1 1/2 c. coconut cream
- 26 oz. chopped celery leaves and stalks
- 1 lb. cubed pork meat
- 1 tbsp. chopped onion

Directions:

1. Heat up a pan while using oil over medium-high heat, add the pork as well as the onion, black pepper and fenugreek, toss and brown for 5 minutes.
2. Add the celery too because coconut cream, toss, cook over medium heat for twenty minutes, divide everything into bowls and serve.
3. Enjoy!

Nutrition:

Calories: 340, Fat:5 g, Carbs:8 g, Protein:14 g, Sugars:2.1 g, Sodium:200 mg

Pork And Dates Sauce

Preparation time: 10 Minutes

Cooking Time: 40 minutes

Servings: 6

Ingredients:

- 2 tbsps. Water
- 2 tbsps. Mustard
- 1/3 c. pitted dates
- Black pepper
- 1/4 tsp. onion powder
- 1/4 c. coconut amino
- 1 1/2 lbs. pork tenderloin
- 1/4 tsp. smoked paprika

Directions:

1. In your blender, mix dates with water, coconut amino, mustard, paprika, pepper and onion powder and blend well.
2. Put pork tenderloin within the roasting pan, add the dates sauce, toss to coat perfectly, introduce everything inside the oven at 400F, bake for 40 minutes, slice the meat, divide it as well since the sauce between plates and serve.
3. Enjoy!

Nutrition:

Calories: 240, Fat: 8 g, Carbs:13 g, Protein:24 g, Sugars: 0 g, Sodium:433 mg

Pork Roast And Cranberry Roast

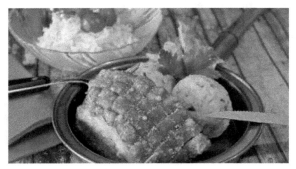

Preparation time: 10 Minutes

Cooking Time: 30 minutes

Servings: 4

Ingredients:

- 2 minced garlic cloves
- 1/2 tsp. grated ginger
- Black pepper
- 1/2 c. low-sodium veggie stock
- 1 1/2 lbs. pork loin roast
- 1 tbsp. coconut flour
- 1/2 c. cranberries
- Juice of 1/2 lemon

Directions:

1. Put the stock in the little pan, get hot over medium-high heat, add black pepper, ginger, garlic, cranberries, fresh freshly squeezed lemon juice along using the flour, whisk well and cook for ten minutes.
2. Put the roast in the pan, add the cranberry sauce at the very top, introduce inside oven and bake at 375F for an hour and 20 minutes.
3. Slice the roast, divide it along using the sauce between plates and serve.
4. Enjoy!

Nutrition:

Calories: 330, Fat:13 g, Carbs:13 g, Protein:25 g, Sugars:7 g, Sodium:150 mg

Easy Pork Chops

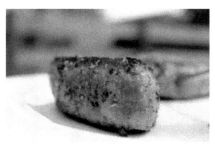

Preparation time: 10 Minutes

Cooking Time: 10 minutes

Servings: 4

Ingredients:

- 1 c. low-sodium chicken stock
- 1 tsp. sweet paprika
- 4 boneless pork chops
- 1/4 tsp. black pepper
- 1 tbsp. extra-virgin olive oil

Directions:

1. Heat up a pan while using the oil over medium-high heat, add pork chops, brown them for 5 minutes on either sides, add paprika, black pepper and stock, toss, cook for fifteen minutes more, divide between plates and serve by using a side salad.
2. Enjoy!

Nutrition:

Calories: 272, Fat:4 g, Carbs:14 g, Protein:17 g, Sugars:0.2 g, Sodium:68 mg

Pork And Roasted Tomatoes Mix

Preparation time: 10 Minutes

Cooking Time: 15 minutes

Servings: 6

Ingredients:

- 1/2 c. chopped yellow onion
- 2 c. chopped zucchinis

- 1 lb. ground pork meat
- ¾ c. shredded low- fat cheddar cheese
- Black pepper
- 15 oz. no-salt-added, chopped and canned roasted tomatoes

Directions:

1. Heat up a pan over medium-high heat, add pork, onion, black pepper and zucchini, stir and cook for 7 minutes.
2. Add roasted tomatoes, stir, bring to a boil, cook over medium heat for 8 minutes, divide into bowls, sprinkle cheddar on the top and serve.
3. Enjoy!

Nutrition:

Calories: 270, Fat:5 g, Carbs:10 g, Protein:12 g, Sugars:8 g, Sodium:390 mg

Provence Pork Medallions

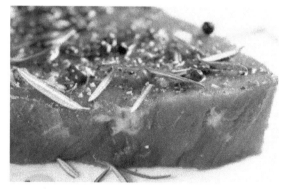

Preparation time: 10 Minutes

Cooking Time: 20 minutes

Servings: 4

Ingredients:

- 1 tsp. Herb de Provence
- Pepper.
- 1/2 c. dry white wine
- 16 oz. pork tenderloins
- Salt

Directions:

1. Season pork lightly with salt and pepper.
2. Place the pork between two pieces of parchment paper and pound with a mallet.
3. You need to have 1/4-inch thick meat.
4. In a large non-stick frying pan, cook the pork over medium-high heat for 2-3 minutes per side.
5. Remove from the heat and sprinkle with herb de Provence. Remove the pork from skillet and place aside. Keep warm.
6. Place the skillet over heat again. Add the wine and cook, stirring to scrape down the bits.
7. Cook until reduced slightly and pour over pork. Serve.

Nutrition:

Calories: 105.7, Fat:1.7 g, Carbs:0.8 g, Protein:22.6 g, Sugars:0 g, Sodium:67 mg

Garlic Pork Shoulder

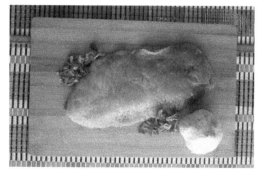

Preparation time: 10 Minutes

Cooking Time: 4 hours

Servings: 6

Ingredients:

- 2 tsps. Sweet paprika
- 4 lbs. pork shoulder

- 3 tbsps. Extra virgin essential olive oil
- Black pepper
- 3 tbsps. Minced garlic

Directions:

1. In a bowl, mix extra virgin extra virgin olive oil with paprika, black pepper and oil and whisk well.
2. Brush pork shoulder with this mix, arrange inside a baking dish and introduce inside oven at 425 0F for twenty or so minutes.

3. Reduce heat to 325 0F F and bake for 4 hours.
4. Slice the meat, divide it between plates and serve having a side salad.
5. Enjoy!

Nutrition:

Calories: 321, Fat:6 g, Carbs:12 g, Protein:18 g, Sugars:0 g, Sodium:470 mg

CHAPTER 12:

Fish And Seafood

Tilapia Tacos With Chipotle Cream

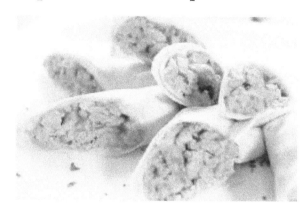

Preparation Time: 5 MINUTES

Cooking Time: 10 MINUTES

Servings: 2

Ingredients:

For the Tacos

- 1 teaspoon olive oil
- 10 to 12 ounces tilapia
- 1 teaspoon chili powder
- 1/2 teaspoon ground cumin
- 1/8 teaspoon salt
- 4 (6-inch) flour tortillas

For the Sauce

- 1/2 teaspoon smoked paprika
- 1/4 teaspoon cayenne pepper, or to taste

- 1/2 cup nonfat Greek yogurt
- 1 chipotle pepper in adobo sauce, chopped

Directions:

To Make the Tacos

1. Heat the oil in a medium skillet on medium-high heat. Add the tilapia to the hot skillet and sprinkle it with the chili powder, cumin, and salt. Cook for 3 to 4 minutes per side. Remove the fish from the heat and gently flake it into bite-size pieces.

2. Wrap the tortillas in a paper towel and heat them for 1 minute in the microwave on high.

To Make the Sauce

3. In a small bowl, mix together the paprika and cayenne pepper. Add the yogurt and chopped chipotle pepper to the spices, blending well.

4. Divide the fish between the tortillas, top with a spoon of the chipotle cream, and serve.

Nutrition: Calories: 383; Total fat: 9g; Carbohydrates: 36g; Fiber: 3g; Protein: 40g; Calcium: 168mg; Sodium: 716mg; Potassium: 727mg; Vitamin D: 2mcg; Iron: 4mg; Zinc: 1mg

Shrimp & Broccoli With Angel Hair

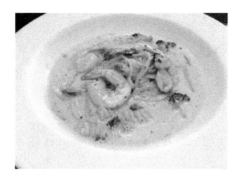

Preparation Time: 10 MINUTES

Cooking Time: 15 MINUTES

Servings: 2

Ingredients:

- Pinch salt

- 4 teaspoons olive oil, divided

- 1 garlic clove, pressed or minced

- 1 broccoli head, cut into florets

- 12 frozen, cooked large shrimp, peeled, deveined, and tails removed

- 4 ounces angel hair pasta

- 2 tablespoons Parmesan cheese

- Freshly ground black pepper (optional)

Directions:

1. Fill a large stockpot three-quarter full with water, adds the salt, and brings it to a boil over high heat.

2. Heat 1 teaspoon of oil in a medium skillet over medium-high heat. Add the garlic and cook for 1 minute. Add the broccoli and sauté for 3 to 4 minutes. Cover and let the vegetables steam for an additional 2 minutes. The broccoli should be bright green and fork-tender. Set aside off the heat.

3. Add the angel hair to the boiling water and cook for 2 to 4 minutes, according to the directions on the package. Drain and immediately add to the skillet. Add the remaining 1 tablespoon of olive oil and stir. Return to low heat to heat through, about 3 minutes.

4. Divide the pasta between two dishes and garnish with the Parmesan cheese and pepper to taste (if using).

Nutrition: Calories: 456; Total fat: 12g; Carbohydrates: 64g; Fiber: 10g; Protein: 25g; Calcium: 230mg; Sodium: 583mg; Potassium: 1158mg; Vitamin D: 0mcg; Iron: 4mg; Zinc: 3mg

Maple-Glazed Salmon

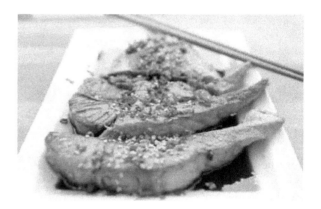

Preparation Time: 15 MINUTES

Cooking Time: 20 MINUTES

Servings: 2

Ingredients:

- 2 (5- to 6-ounce) salmon fillets, skin-on

- 1/2 teaspoon salt-free mesquite seasoning

- 1 tablespoon pure maple syrup

Directions:

1. Preheat the oven to 425°F. Line a baking sheet with parchment paper or a silicone mat. 2. Place the salmon onto the baking sheet (skin side down) and rub the seasoning evenly over each fillet. Drizzle the syrup onto the fillets, rubbing to coat the top.

3. Put the baking sheet in the oven and bake for 15 to 20 minutes. 4. Serve.

Nutrition: Calories: 223; Total fat: 9g; Carbohydrates: 7g; Fiber: 0g; Protein: 28g; Calcium: 27mg; Sodium: 64mg; Potassium: 716mg; Vitamin D: 9mcg; Iron: 1mg; Zinc: 1mg

Marinated Lime Grilled Shrimp

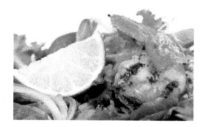

Preparation Time: 10 MINUTES, PLUS AT LEAST 30 MINUTES TO MARINATE Cooking Time: 10 MINUTES

Servings: 2

Ingredients:

- 1 lime, quartered, divided

- 1/4 cup chopped fresh cilantro, divided

- 1 tablespoon rice wine vinegar

- 1 teaspoon avocado oil

- 1/4 teaspoon chili powder

- 1/4 teaspoon garlic powder

- 6 large shrimp, peeled and deveined

Directions:

1. In a small bowl, mix together the juice from three lime quarters, 3 tablespoons cilantro, and the vinegar, oil, chili powder, and garlic powder.

2. Place the shrimp in the bowl with the marinade, toss to coat, and refrigerate it for 30 minutes or up to 4 hours.

3. Preheat a grill to medium-high. Place the shrimp on a grill pan and cook for 3 to 5 minutes, until white, turning once. Discard the marinade. 4. If you do not have a grill, pan-sear the shrimp in a nonstick skillet for 3 to 4 minutes, turning once. 5. Serve the shrimp with a squeeze of juice from the last lime quarter and the remaining cilantro.

Nutrition: Calories: 44; Total fat: 2g; Carbohydrates: 3g; Fiber: 0g; Protein: 3g; Calcium: 18mg; Sodium: 131mg; Potassium: 74mg; Vitamin D: 0mcg; Iron: 0 mg; Zinc: 0mg

Angel Hair With Smoked Salmon & Asparagus

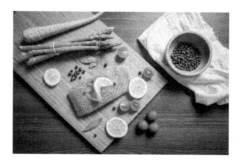

Preparation Time: 15 MINUTES

Cooking Time: 15 MINUTES

Servings: 2

Ingredients:

- 20 asparagus spears, trimmed and cut into 2-inch pieces

- 2 tablespoons olive oil, divided

- 4 ounces angel hair pasta

- 2 ounces smoked salmon, cut into bite-size pieces

- 1 teaspoon capers

- 2 tablespoons grated Parmesan cheese

- Freshly ground black pepper

Directions:

1. Fill a large stockpot three-quarters full with water and bring it to a boil over high heat.

2. Add 2 tablespoons of water to a large nonstick skillet over medium heat. When the water is simmering, add the asparagus, cover, and steam for 6 minutes. Remove the lid, drain off any remaining water, and add 11/2 teaspoons oil, and sauté for 1 to 2 more minutes.

3. Add the angel hair pasta to the boiling water and cook for 3 minutes (or according to the package directions). Drain the pasta, transfer it to a serving bowl, and add the asparagus, smoked salmon, the remaining 11/2 tablespoons oil, and the capers and toss gently.

4. Serve topped with the Parmesan cheese and season to taste with pepper.

Nutrition: Calories: 416; Total fat: 17g; Carbohydrates: 49g; Fiber: 5g; Protein: 18g; Calcium: 97mg; Sodium: 320mg; Potassium: 509mg; Vitamin D: 5mcg; Iron: 6mg; Zinc: 2mg

Bass With Citrus Butter

Preparation Time: 15 MINUTES

Cooking Time: 15 MINUTES

Servings: 2

Ingredients:

- 2 (5- to 7-ounce) bass fillets, skin-on

- 1 teaspoon salt-free seafood seasoning

- 1/8 teaspoon salt

- 1 lime, halved

- 1 tablespoon avocado oil, divided

- 1 teaspoon butter

- 1/4 teaspoon cumin

- 1/4 cup slivered, blanched almonds

Directions:

1. Season the fish with the seasoning blend and salt. 2. In a microwave-safe glass measuring cup, stir together the juice of half a lime, 2 teaspoons oil, butter, and cumin until blended. Set aside.

3. Heat a large nonstick skillet over medium heat. Add the almonds and toast for 2 to 3 minutes, being careful they don't over-brown. Transfer the almonds to a small bowl and set aside.

4. Heat the remaining oil in the skillet over medium-high heat. Add the bass fillets, skin side up. Sear for 3 minutes without disturbing the fillets, then turn them and finish cooking for another 3 to 4 minutes.

5. While the fish is searing, heat the citrus butter sauce for 20 seconds in the microwave. 6. Transfer the fish to a serving dish, pour the citrus butter over it, and top it with the toasted almonds. Garnish with the remaining lime half cut into wedges and serve.

Nutrition: Calories: 325; Total fat: 21g; Carbohydrates: 5g; Fiber: 2g; Protein: 30g; Calcium: 156mg; Sodium: 270mg; Potassium: 634mg; Vitamin D: 13mcg; Iron: 3mg; Zinc: 1mg

Seared Mahi-Mahi With Lemon & Parsley

Preparation Time: 20 MINUTES, PLUS AT LEAST 15 MINUTES TO MARINATE
Cooking Time: 15 MINUTES

Servings: 2

Ingredients:

- 2 teaspoons avocado oil

- Juice of 1/2 lemon

- 1/2 teaspoon oregano

- 1/2 teaspoon garlic powder

- 1/4 teaspoon Worcestershire sauce

- 2 (5- to 7-ounce) mahi-mahi steaks

- 1 tablespoon chopped parsley

- 1/2 lemon, cut into two wedges

Directions:

1. Preheat the oven to 400°F. (If you'll be marinating the fish for longer than 15 minutes, preheat the oven just before baking.) Line a baking sheet with parchment paper or a silicone mat.

2. In a medium bowl, stir together the oil, lemon juice, oregano, garlic powder, and Worcestershire sauce. Put the fish in a medium zip-top plastic bag and add the marinade. Press out any excess air, seal the bag, and marinate the fish in the refrigerator for 15 minutes or up to 2 hours.

3. Remove the fish from the marinade, place it on the prepared baking sheet, and roast it for 15 minutes (discard the marinade).

4. To serve, garnish each mahi-mahi steak with parsley and a lemon wedge.

Nutrition: Calories: 282; Total fat: 18g; Carbohydrates: 3g; Fiber: g; Protein: 26g; Calcium: 41mg; Sodium: 101mg; Potassium: 594mg; Vitamin D: 16mcg; Iron: 1mg; Zinc: 1mg

Pan-Fried Crusted Salmon With Mustard Panko

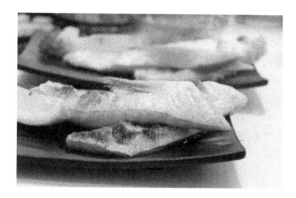

Preparation Time: 5 MINUTES

Cooking Time: 10 MINUTES

Servings: 2

Ingredients:

- 1 tablespoon Dijon mustard

- 1 tablespoon light sour cream

- 2 skinless salmon fillets (5 to 6 ounces each)

- 1/4 cup panko bread crumbs

- 1/2 teaspoon salt-free mesquite seasoning

- 1 teaspoon olive oil

- 1 teaspoon butter

Directions:

1. In a small bowl, combine the mustard and sour cream. Spread the mustard mixture onto both sides of each salmon fillet, dividing evenly between the two.

2. Mix the panko bread crumbs and seasoning together in a small bowl. Press each fillet into the seasoned crumbs, lightly coating both sides.

3. Heat the oil and butter in a large nonstick skillet over medium-high heat. Place the fish into the hot fat to fry. Gently turn each fillet after 4 to 5 minutes, and pan-fry the other side for another 5 to 6 minutes until lightly browned. The salmon should change to a lighter color but not be opaque. Serve hot.

Nutrition: Calories: 307; Total fat: 15g; Carbohydrates: 11g; Fiber: 1g; Protein: 31g; Calcium: 56mg; Sodium: 689mg; Potassium: 746mg; Vitamin D: 9mcg; Iron: 2mg; Zinc: 1mg

Seared Ginger–Soy Ahi Tuna

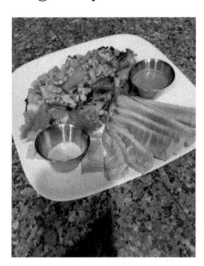

Preparation Time: 10 MINUTES

Cooking Time: 2 MINUTES

Servings: 2

Ingredients:

- 2 tablespoons reduced-sodium soy sauce, divided

- Juice of 1 lime

- 2 teaspoons Dijon mustard

- 1/4 teaspoon ground ginger

- 10 ounces sushi-grade tuna

- 1 teaspoon olive oil

- 4 scallions, both white and green parts, thinly sliced

Directions:

1. In a small bowl, mix together 1 tablespoon of the soy sauce with the lime juice, mustard, and ginger until blended. Using a basting brush, brush the mixture onto each side of the tuna.

2. Heat the oil in a large nonstick skillet over high heat. Add the tuna, searing one side for 1 minute. Flip the fish over and sear the other side for 1 minute. The fish should still be pink in the middle.

3. Remove the tuna from the skillet, transfer it to a small serving platter, and cut it on the diagonal into 1/4-inch slices. Top with the scallions and serve with the remaining soy sauce.

Nutrition: Calories: 126; Total fat: 5g; Carbohydrates: 3g; Fiber: 1g; Protein: 18g; Calcium: 22mg; Sodium: 313mg; Potassium: 263mg; Vitamin D: 4mcg; Iron: 1mg; Zinc: 1mg

Greek-Style Cod With Olives & Tomatoes

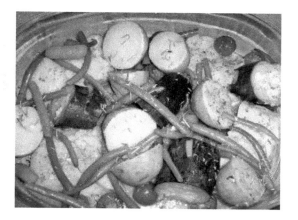

Preparation Time: 15 MINUTES

Cooking Time: 35 MINUTES

Servings: 2

Ingredients:

- 1 pint grape or cherry tomatoes, halved

- ⅓ cup mixed olives, pitted, roughly chopped

- 1 teaspoon olive oil

- 2 cod fillets (5 to 8 ounces each)

- 1 teaspoon Herbs de Provence

- 2 lemon wedges, for garnish

Directions:

1. Preheat the oven to 375°F. Line a baking sheet with parchment paper or a silicone mat.

2. Place the tomatoes and olives on one half of the baking sheet and drizzle them with olive oil. Roast in the oven for 15 minutes.

3. Remove the baking sheet from the oven, place the cod fillets on the empty side, and season both the tomato mixture and the fish with Herbs de Provence. Bake for 15 to 20 minutes until the fish is opaque.

4. Serve the fish topped with the olive-tomato mixture and garnished with a squeeze of lemon.

Nutrition: Calories: 186; Total fat: 6g; Carbohydrates: 8g; Fiber: 2g; Protein: 26g; Calcium: 53mg; Sodium: 244mg; Potassium: 813mg; Vitamin D: 1mcg; Iron: 2mg; Zinc: 1mg

Pesto Tilapia

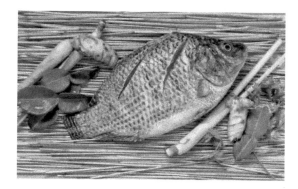

Preparation Time: 5 MINUTES

Cooking Time: 20 MINUTES

Servings: 2

Ingredients:

- 1/4 cup dry white wine

- 1 teaspoon avocado oil

- 1 lemon, halved

- 2 tilapia fillets (5 to 7 ounces each)

- Freshly ground black pepper

- 2 tablespoons store-bought low-sodium pesto

Directions:

1. Preheat the oven to 350°F.

2. In a 9-by-11-inch baking dish, whisk the wine, oil, and juice of half a lemon. Add the fish fillets and season lightly with pepper.

3. Cover the baking dish with foil and bake for 15 minutes. Uncover the dish, top each fillet with 1 tablespoon pesto, and cook for 5 more minutes.

4. Cut the remaining 1/2 lemon into wedges and serve each fillet with a lemon wedge.

Nutrition: Calories: 272; Total fat: 13g; Carbohydrates: 3g; Fiber: 0g; Protein: 30g; Calcium: 56mg; Sodium: 220mg; Potassium: 502mg; Vitamin D: 4mcg; Iron: 1mg; Zinc: 1mg

CHAPTER 13:

Vegan And Vegetarian

Spinach Dip

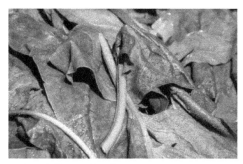

Preparation Time: 4 minutes

Cooking Time: 0 minutes

Servings: 2

Ingredients:

- 5 ounces Spinach, raw
- 1 cup Greek yogurt
- 1/2 tablespoon onion powder
- 1/4 teaspoon garlic sunflower seeds
- Black pepper to taste
- 1/4 teaspoon Greek Seasoning

Directions:

1. Add the listed ingredients in a blender.

2. Emulsify.

3. Season and serve.

Nutrition:

Calories: 101 Fat: 4g

Carbohydrates: 4g

Protein: 10g

Cauliflower Rice

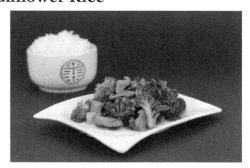

Preparation Time: 5 minutes

Cooking Time: 6 minutes

Servings: 2

Ingredients:

- 1 head grated cauliflower head
- 1 tablespoon coconut amino
- 1 pinch of sunflower seeds
- 1 pinch of black pepper
- 1 tablespoon Garlic Powder
- 1 tablespoon Sesame Oil

Directions:

1. Add cauliflower to a food processor and grate it.

2. Take a pan and add sesame oil, let it heat up over medium heat.

3. Add grated cauliflower and pour coconut amino. Cook for 4-6 minutes. Season and enjoy!

Nutrition:

Calories: 329 Fat: 28g Carbohydrates: 13g

Protein: 10g

Grilled Sprouts And Balsamic Glaze

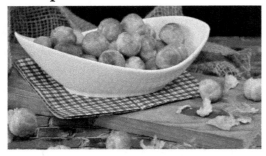

Preparation Time: 10 minutes

Cooking Time: 30 minutes

Servings: 2

Ingredients:

- 1/2 pound Brussels sprouts, trimmed and halved
- Fresh cracked black pepper
- 1 tablespoon olive oil
- Sunflower seeds to taste
- 2 teaspoons balsamic glaze
- 2 wooden skewers

Directions:

1. Take wooden skewers and place them on a largely sized foil.
2. Place sprouts on the skewers and drizzle oil, sprinkle sunflower seeds and pepper.
3. Cover skewers with foil.
4. Pre-heat your grill to low and place skewers (with foil) in the grill.
5. Grill for 30 minutes, making sure to turn after every 5-6 minutes.
6. Once done, uncovered and drizzle balsamic glaze on top.
7. Enjoy!

Nutrition:

Calories: 440 Fat: 27g

Carbohydrates: 33g Protein: 26g

Amazing Green Creamy Cabbage

Preparation Time: 10 minutes

Cooking Time: 10 minutes

Servings: 4

Ingredients:

- 2 ounces almond butter
- 1 1/2 pounds green cabbage, shredded
- 1 1/4 cups coconut cream
- Sunflower seeds and pepper to taste
- 8 tablespoons fresh parsley, chopped

Directions:

1. Take a skillet and place it over medium heat, add almond butter and let it melt.
2. Add cabbage and sauté until brown.
3. Stir in cream and lower the heat to low.
4. Let it simmer.
5. Season with sunflower seeds and pepper.
6. Garnish with parsley and serve.
7. Enjoy!

Nutrition:

Calories: 432 Fat: 42g

Carbohydrates: 8g Protein: 4g

Simple Rice Mushroom Risotto

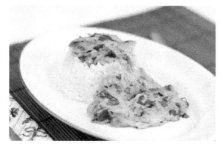

Preparation Time: 5 minutes

Cooking Time: 15 minutes

Servings: 4

Ingredients:

- 4 1/2 cups cauliflower, riced

- 3 tablespoons coconut oil

- 1 pound Portobello mushrooms, thinly sliced

- 1 pound white mushrooms, thinly sliced

- 2 shallots, diced

- 1/4 cup organic vegetable broth

- Sunflower seeds and pepper to taste

- 3 tablespoons chives, chopped

- 4 tablespoons almond butter

- 1/2 cup kite ricotta/cashew cheese, grated

Directions:

1. Use a food processor and pulse cauliflower florets until riced.

2. Take a large saucepan and heat up 2 tablespoons oil over medium-high flame.

3. Add mushrooms and sauté for 3 minutes until mushrooms are tender.

4. Clear saucepan of mushrooms and liquid and keep them on the side.

5. Add the rest of the 1 tablespoon oil to skillet.

6. Toss shallots and cook for 60 seconds.

7. Add cauliflower rice, stir for 2 minutes until coated with oil.

8. Add broth to riced cauliflower and stir for 5 minutes.

9. Remove pot from heat and mix in mushrooms and liquid.

10. Add chives, almond butter, and parmesan cheese.

11. Season with sunflower seeds and pepper. Serve and enjoy!

Nutrition:

Calories: 438 Fat: 17g Carbohydrates: 15g

Protein: 12g

Hearty Green Bean Roast

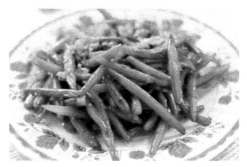

Preparation Time: 10 minutes

Cooking Time: 20 minutes

Servings: 4

Ingredients:

- 1 whole egg

- 2 tablespoons olive oil

- Sunflower seeds and pepper to taste

- 1 pound fresh green beans

- 5 1/2 tablespoons grated parmesan cheese

Directions:

1. Pre-heat your oven to 400 degrees F.

2. Take a bowl and whisk in eggs with oil and spices. Add beans and mix well.

3. Stir in parmesan cheese and pour the mix into baking pan (lined with parchment paper). Bake for 15-20 minutes.

4. Serve warm and enjoy!

Nutrition:

Calories: 216 Fat: 21g Carbohydrates: 7g

Protein: 9g

Almond And Blistered Beans

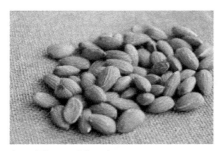

Preparation Time: 10 minutes

Cooking Time: 20 minutes

Servings: 4

Ingredients:

- 1 pound fresh green beans, ends trimmed

- 1 1/2 tablespoon olive oil

- 1/4 teaspoon sunflower seeds

- 1 1/2 tablespoons fresh dill, minced

- Juice of 1 lemon

- 1/4 cup crushed almonds

- Sunflower seeds as needed

Directions:

1. Pre-heat your oven to 400 degrees F. Add the green beans with your olive oil and also the sunflower seeds.

2. Then spread them in one single layer on a large sized sheet pan.

3. Roast it for 10 minutes and stir, then roast for another 8-10 minutes.

4. Remove from the oven and keep stirring in the lemon juice alongside the dill. Top it with crushed almonds and some flaked sunflower seeds and serve.

Nutrition:

Calories: 347 Fat: 16g Carbohydrates: 6g

Protein: 45g

Tomato Platter

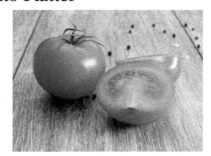

Preparation Time: 10 minutes + Chill time

Cooking Time: 0

Servings: 8

Ingredients:

- 1/3 cup olive oil

- 1 teaspoon sunflower seeds
- 2 tablespoons onion, chopped
- 1/4 teaspoon pepper
- 1/2 a garlic, minced
- 1 tablespoon fresh parsley, minced
- 3 large fresh tomatoes, sliced
- 1 teaspoon dried basil
- 1/4 cup red wine vinegar

Directions:

1. Take a shallow dish and arrange tomatoes in the dish.
2. Add the rest of the ingredients in a mason jar, cover the jar and shake it well.
3. Pour the mix over tomato slices.
4. Let it chill for 2-3 hours.
5. Serve!

Nutrition:

Calories: 350

Fat: 28g

Carbohydrates: 10g

Protein: 14g

Lemony Sprouts

Preparation Time: 10 minutes

Cooking Time: 0

Servings: 4

Ingredients:

- 1 pound Brussels sprouts, trimmed and shredded
- 8 tablespoons olive oil

- 1 lemon, juice and zested
- Sunflower seeds and pepper to taste
- ¾ cup spicy almond and seed mix

Directions:

1. Take a bowl and mix in lemon juice, sunflower seeds, pepper and olive oil.
2. Mix well.
3. Stir in shredded Brussels sprouts and toss.
4. Let it sit for 10 minutes.
5. Add nuts and toss.
6. Serve and enjoy!

Nutrition:

Calories: 382

Fat: 36g

Carbohydrates: 9g

Protein: 7g

Cool Garbanzo And Spinach Beans

Preparation Time: 5-10 minutes

Cooking Time: 0

Servings: 4

Ingredients:

- 1 tablespoon olive oil
- 1/2 onion, diced
- 10 ounces spinach, chopped
- 12 ounces garbanzo beans
- 1/2 teaspoon cumin

Directions:

1. Take a skillet and add olive oil, let it warm over medium-low heat.
2. Add onions, garbanzo and cook for 5 minutes.

3. Stir in spinach, cumin, garbanzo beans and season with sunflower seeds.

4. Use a spoon to smash gently.

5. Cook thoroughly until heated, enjoys!

Nutrition:

Calories: 90

Fat: 4g

Carbohydrates:11g

Protein:4g

Delicious Garlic Tomatoes

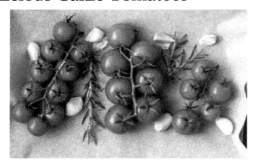

Preparation Time: 10 minutes

Cooking Time: 50 minutes

Servings: 4

Ingredients:

- 4 garlic cloves, crushed
- 1 pound mixed cherry tomatoes
- 3 thyme sprigs, chopped
- Pinch of sunflower seeds
- Black pepper as needed
- 1/4 cup olive oil

Directions:

1. Preheat your oven to 325 degrees F.

2. Take a baking dish and add tomatoes, olive oil and thyme.

3. Season with sunflower seeds and pepper and mix.

4. Bake for 50 minutes.

5. Divide tomatoes and pan juices and serve.

6. Enjoy!

Nutrition:

Calories: 100

Fat: 0g

Carbohydrates: 1g

Protein: 6g

Mashed Celeriac

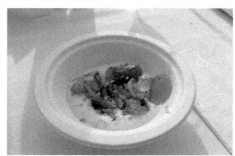

Preparation Time: 10 minutes

Cooking Time: 20 minutes

Servings: 4

Ingredients:

- 2 celeriac, washed, peeled and diced
- 2 teaspoons extra-virgin olive oil
- 1 tablespoon honey
- 1/2 teaspoon ground nutmeg
- Sunflower seeds and pepper as needed

Directions:

1. Pre-heat your oven to 400 degrees F.

2. Line a baking sheet with aluminum foil and keep it on the side.

3. Take a large bowl and toss celeriac and olive oil.

4. Spread celeriac evenly on a baking sheet.

5. Roast for 20 minutes until tender.

6. Transfer to a large bowl.

7. Add honey and nutmeg.

8. Use a potato masher to mash the mixture until fluffy.

9. Season with sunflower seeds and pepper.

10. Serve and enjoy!

Nutrition:

Calories: 136

Fat: 3g

Carbohydrates: 26g

Protein: 4g

Spicy Wasabi Mayonnaise

Preparation Time: 15 minutes

Cooking Time: 0

Servings: 4

Ingredients:

- 1 cup mayonnaise
- 1/2 tablespoon wasabi paste

Directions:

1. Take a bowl and mix wasabi paste and mayonnaise.

2. Mix well.

3. Let it chill and use as needed.

Nutrition:

Calories: 388 Fat: 42g Carbohydrates: 1g

Protein: 1g

Mediterranean Kale Dish

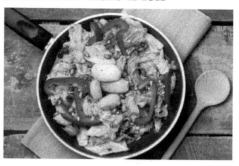

Preparation Time: 15 minutes

Cooking Time: 10 minutes

Servings: 6

Ingredients:

- 12 cups kale, chopped
- 2 tablespoons lemon juice
- 1 tablespoon olive oil
- 1 teaspoon coconut amino
- Sunflower seeds and pepper as needed

Directions:

1. Add a steamer insert to your saucepan.

2. Fill the saucepan with water up to the bottom of the steamer.

3. Cover and bring water to boil (medium-high heat).

4. Add kale to the insert and steam for 7-8 minutes.

5. Take a large bowl and add lemon juice, olive oil, sunflower seeds, coconut amino, and pepper.

6. Mix well and add the steamed kale to the bowl. Toss and serve. Enjoy!

Nutrition:

Calories: 350 Fat: 17g Carbohydrates: 41g

Protein: 11g

Spicy Kale Chips

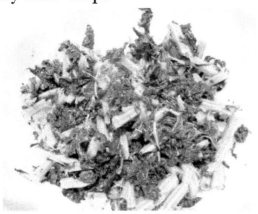

Preparation Time: 10 minutes

Cooking Time: 25 minutes

Servings: 4

Ingredients:

- 3 cups kale, stemmed and thoroughly washed, torn in 2-inch pieces
- 1 tablespoon extra-virgin olive oil
- 1/2 teaspoon chili powder
- 1/4 teaspoon salted sunflower seeds

Directions:

1. Pre-heat your oven to 300 degrees F.

2. Line 2 baking sheets with parchment paper and keep it on the side.

3. Dry kale entirely and transfer to a large bowl.

4. Add olive oil and toss.

5. Make sure each leaf is covered.

6. Season kale with chili powder and sunflower seeds, toss again.

7. Divide kale between baking sheets and spread into a single layer.

8. Bake for 25 minutes until crispy.

9. Cool the chips for 5 minutes and serve.

10. Enjoy!

Nutrition:

Calories: 56

Fat: 4g

Carbohydrates: 5g

Protein: 2g

Seemingly Easy Portobello Mushrooms

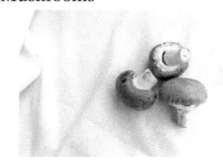

Preparation Time: 10 minutes

Cooking Time: 10 minutes

Servings: 4

Ingredients:

- 12 cherry tomatoes
- 2 ounces scallions
- 4 portabella mushrooms
- 4 1/4 ounces almond butter
- Sunflower seeds and pepper to taste

Directions:

1. Take a large skillet and melt almond butter over medium heat.

2. Add mushrooms and sauté for 3 minutes.

3. Stir in cherry tomatoes and scallions.

4. Sauté for 5 minutes.

5. Season accordingly.

6. Sauté until veggies are tender.

7. Enjoy!

Nutrition:

Calories: 154

Fat: 10g

Carbohydrates: 2g

Protein: 7g

The Garbanzo Bean Extravaganza

Preparation Time: 10 minutes

Cooking Time: 20 minutes

Servings: 5

Ingredients:

- 1 can garbanzo beans, chickpeas
- 1 tablespoon olive oil
- 1 teaspoon sunflower seeds
- 1 teaspoon garlic powder
- 1/2 teaspoon paprika

Directions:

1. Pre-heat your oven to 375 degrees F.

2. Line a baking sheet with a silicone baking mat.

3. Drain and rinse garbanzo beans, pat garbanzo beans dry and put into a large bowl.

4. Toss with olive oil, sunflower seeds, garlic powder, and paprika and mix well.

5. Spread over a baking sheet.

6. Bake for 20 minutes.

7. Turn chickpeas so they are roasted well.

8. Place back in oven and bake for another 25 minutes at 375 degrees F.

9. Let them cool and enjoy!

Nutrition:

Calories: 395

Fat: 7g

Carbohydrates: 52g

Protein: 35g

CHAPTER 14:

Desserts

Mesmerizing Avocado And Chocolate Pudding

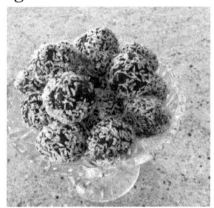

Preparation Time: 30 minutes

Cooking Time: 0 minutes

Servings: 2

Ingredients:

- 1 avocado, chunked
- 1 tablespoon natural sweetener such as stevia
- 2 ounces cream cheese, at room temp
- 1/4 teaspoon vanilla extract
- 4 tablespoons cocoa powder, unsweetened

Directions:

1. Blend listed ingredients in blender until smooth.
2. Divide the mix between dessert bowls, chill for 30 minutes.
3. Serve and enjoy!

Nutrition:

Calories: 281 Fat: 27g Carbohydrates: 12g

Protein: 8g

Hearty Pineapple Pudding

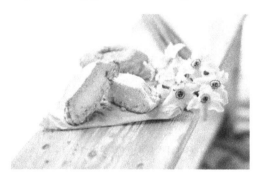

Preparation Time: 10 minutes

Cooking Time: 5 hours

Servings: 4

Ingredients:

- 1 teaspoon baking powder
- 1 cup coconut flour
- 3 tablespoons stevia
- 3 tablespoons avocado oil
- 1/2 cup coconut milk
- 1/2 cup pecans, chopped
- 1/2 cup pineapple, chopped
- 1/2 cup lemon zest, grated
- 1 cup pineapple juice, natural

Directions:

1. Grease Slow Cooker with oil.

2. Take a bowl and mix in flour, stevia, baking powder, oil, milk, pecans, pineapple, lemon zest, pineapple juice and stir well.

3. Pour the mix into the Slow Cooker.

4. Place lid and cook on LOW for 5 hours.

5. Divide between bowls and serve.

6. Enjoy!

Nutrition:

Calories: 188 Fat: 3g

Carbohydrates: 14g Protein: 5g

Healthy Berry Cobbler

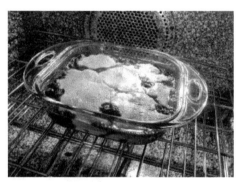

Preparation Time: 10 minutes

Cooking Time: 2 hours 30 minutes

Servings: 8

Ingredients:

- 1 1/4 cups almond flour
- 1 cup coconut sugar
- 1 teaspoon baking powder
- 1/2 teaspoon cinnamon powder
- 1 whole egg
- 1/4 cup low-fat milk
- 2 tablespoons olive oil
- 2 cups raspberries
- 2 cups blueberries

Directions:

1. Take a bowl and add almond flour, coconut sugar, baking powder and cinnamon.

2. Stir well .

3. Take another bowl and add egg, milk, oil, raspberries, blueberries and stir.

4. Combine both of the mixtures.

5. Grease your Slow Cooker.

6. Pour the combined mixture into your Slow Cooker and cook on HIGH for 2 hours 30 minutes.

7. Divide between serving bowls and enjoy!

Nutrition:

Calories: 250 Fat: 4g

Carbohydrates: 30g Protein: 3g

Tasty Poached Apples

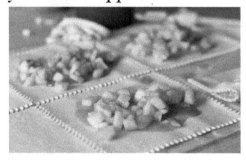

Preparation Time: 10 minutes

Cooking Time: 2 hours 30 minutes

Servings: 8

Ingredients:

- 6 apples, cored, peeled and sliced
- 1 cup apple juice, natural
- 1 cup coconut sugar
- 1 tablespoon cinnamon powder

Directions:

1. Grease Slow Cooker with cooking spray.
2. Add apples, sugar, juice, cinnamon to your Slow Cooker.
3. Stir gently.
4. Place lid and cook on HIGH for 4 hours. Serve cold and enjoy!

Nutrition:

Calories: 180 Fat: 5g

Carbohydrates: 8g Protein: 4g

Apple And Almond Muffins

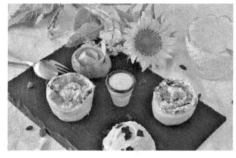

Preparation Time: 10 minutes

Cooking Time: 20 minutes

Servings: 6 muffins

Ingredients:

- 6 ounces ground almonds
- 1 teaspoon cinnamon
- 1/2 teaspoon baking powder
- 1 pinch sunflower seeds
- 1 whole egg
- 1 teaspoon apple cider vinegar
- 2 tablespoons Erythritol
- 1/3 cup apple sauce

Directions:

1. Pre-heat your oven to 350 degrees F.
2. Line muffin tin with paper muffin cups, keep them on the side.
3. Mix in almonds, cinnamon, baking powder, sunflower seeds and keep it on the side.
4. Take another bowl and beat in eggs, apple cider vinegar, apple sauce, Erythritol.
5. Add the mix to dry ingredients and mix well until you have a smooth batter.
6. Pour batter into tin and bake for 20 minutes.
7. Once done, let them cool.
8. Serve and enjoy!

Nutrition:

Total Carbs: 10 Fiber: 4g Protein: 13g Fat: 17g

Stylish Chocolate Parfait

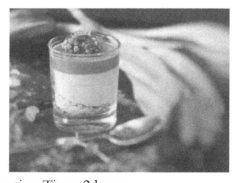

Preparation Time: 2 hours

Cooking Time: 0 minutes

Servings: 4

Ingredients:

- 2 tablespoons cocoa powder
- 1 cup almond milk

- 1 tablespoon chia seeds
- Pinch of sunflower seeds
- 1/2 teaspoon vanilla extract

Directions:

1. Take a bowl and add cocoa powder, almond milk, chia seeds, va0 mensal extract and stir.

2. Transfer to dessert glass and place in your fridge for 2 hours.

3. Serve and enjoy!

Nutrition:

Calories: 130

Fat: 5g

Carbohydrates: 7g

Protein: 16g

Supreme Matcha Bomb

Preparation Time: 100 minutes

Cooking Time: 0 minutes

Servings: 10

Ingredients:

- 3/4 cup hemp seeds
- 1/2 cup coconut oil
- 2 tablespoons coconut almond butter
- 1 teaspoon Matcha powder
- 2 tablespoons vanilla bean extract
- 1/2 teaspoon mint extract
- Liquid stevia

Directions:

1. Take your blender/food processor and add hemp seeds, coconut oil,

Matcha, va0 mensal extract and stevia.

2. Blend until you have a nice batter and divide into silicon molds.

3. Melt coconut almond butter and drizzle on top.

4. Let the cups chill and enjoy!

Nutrition:

Calories: 200

Fat: 20g

Carbohydrates: 3g

Protein: 5g

Home Made Trail Mix For The Trip

Preparation Time: 10 minutes

Cooking Time: 55 minutes

Servings: 4

Ingredients:

- 1/4 cup raw cashews
- 1/4 cup almonds
- 1/4 cup walnuts
- 1 teaspoon cinnamon
- 2 tablespoons melted coconut oil
- Sunflower seeds as needed

Directions:

1. Line baking sheet with parchment paper.

2. Pre-heat your oven to 275 degrees F.

3. Melt coconut oil and keep it on the side.

4. Combine nuts to large mixing bowl and add cinnamon and melted coconut oil.

5. Stir.

6. Sprinkle sunflower seeds.

7. Place in oven and brown for 6 minutes.

8. Enjoy!

Nutrition:

Calories: 363

Fat: 22g

Carbohydrates: 41g

Protein: 7g

Heart Warming Cinnamon Rice Pudding

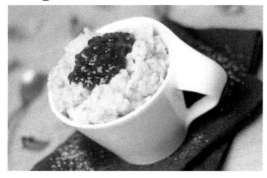

Preparation Time: 10 minutes

Cooking Time: 5 hours

Servings: 4

Ingredients:

- 6 1/2 cups water
- 1 cup coconut sugar
- 2 cups white rice
- 2 cinnamon sticks
- 1/2 cup coconut, shredded

Directions:

1. Add water, rice, sugar, cinnamon and coconut to your Slow Cooker.

2. Gently stir.

3. Place lid and cook on HIGH for 5 hours.

4. Discard cinnamon.

5. Divide pudding between dessert dishes and enjoy!

Nutrition:

Calories: 173

Fat: 4g

Carbohydrates: 9g

Protein: 4g

Pure Avocado Pudding

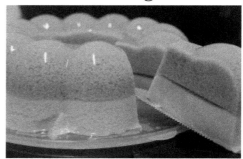

Preparation Time: 3 hours

Cooking Time: 0 minutes

Servings: 4

Ingredients:

- 1 cup almond milk
- 2 avocados, peeled and pitted
- ¾ cup cocoa powder
- 1 teaspoon vanilla extract
- 2 tablespoons stevia
- 1/4 teaspoon cinnamon
- Walnuts, chopped for serving

Directions:

1. Add avocados to a blender and pulse well.

2. Add cocoa powder, almond milk, stevia, vanilla bean extract and pulse the mixture well.

3. Pour into serving bowls and top with walnuts.

4. Chill for 2-3 hours and serve!

Nutrition:

Calories: 221

Fat: 8g

Carbohydrates: 7g

Protein: 3g

Sweet Almond And Coconut Fat Bombs

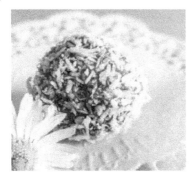

Preparation Time: 10 minutes

Cooking Time: 0

Freeze Time: 20 minutes

Servings: 6

Ingredients:

- 1/4 cup melted coconut oil

- 9 1/2 tablespoons almond butter

- 90 drops liquid stevia

- 3 tablespoons cocoa

- 9 tablespoons melted almond butter, sunflower seeds

Directions:

1. Take a bowl and add all of the listed ingredients.

2. Mix them well.

3. Pour 2 tablespoons of the mixture into as many muffin molds as you like.

4. Chill for 20 minutes and pop them out.

5. Serve and enjoy!

Nutrition:

Total Carbs: 2g

Fiber: 0g

Protein: 2.53g

Fat: 14g

Spicy Popper Mug Cake

Preparation Time: 5 minutes

Cooking Time: 5 minutes

Servings: 2

Ingredients:

- 2 tablespoons almond flour

- 1 tablespoon flaxseed meal

- 1 tablespoon almond butter

- 1 tablespoon cream cheese

- 1 large egg

- 1 bacon, cooked and sliced

- 1/2 jalapeno pepper

- 1/2 teaspoon baking powder

- 1/4 teaspoon sunflower seeds

Directions:

1. Take a frying pan and place it over medium heat.

2. Add slice of bacon and cook until it has a crispy texture.

3. Take a microwave proof container and mix all of the listed ingredients (including cooked bacon), clean the sides.

4. Microwave for 75 seconds, making to put your microwave to high power.

5. Take out the cup and tap it against a surface to take the cake out.

6. Garnish with a bit of jalapeno and serve!

Nutrition:

Calories: 429

Fat: 38g

Carbohydrates: 6g

Protein: 16g

The Most Elegant Parsley Soufflé Ever

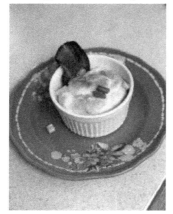

Preparation Time: 5 minutes

Cooking Time: 6 minutes

Servings: 5

Ingredients:

- 2 whole eggs

- 1 fresh red chili pepper, chopped

- 2 tablespoons coconut cream

- 1 tablespoon fresh parsley, chopped

- Sunflower seeds to taste

Directions:

1. Pre-heat your oven to 390 degrees F.

2. Almond butter 2 soufflé dishes.

3. Add the ingredients to a blender and mix well.

4. Divide batter into soufflé dishes and bake for 6 minutes.

5. Serve and enjoy!

Nutrition:

Calories: 108 Fat: 9g Carbohydrates: 9g

Protein: 6g

Fennel And Almond Bites

Preparation Time: 10 minutes

Cooking Time: None

Freeze Time: 3 hours

Servings: 12

Ingredients:

- 1 teaspoon vanilla extract

- 1/4 cup almond milk

- 1/4 cup cocoa powder

- 1/2 cup almond oil

- A pinch of sunflower seeds

- 1 teaspoon fennel seeds

Directions:

1. Take a bowl and mix the almond oil and almond milk.

2. Beat until smooth and glossy using electric beater.

3. Mix in the rest of the ingredients.

4. Take a piping bag and pour into a parchment paper lined baking sheet.

5. Freeze for 3 hours and store in the fridge.

Nutrition:

Total Carbs: 1g   Fiber: 1g Protein: 1g   Fat: 20g

Feisty Coconut Fudge

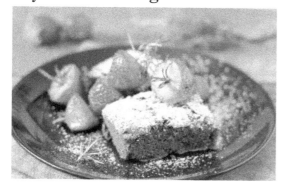

Preparation Time: 20 minutes

Cooking Time: None

Freeze Time: 2 hours

Servings: 12

Ingredients:

- 1/4 cup coconut, shredded

- 2 cups coconut oil

- 1/2 cup coconut cream

- 1/4 cup almonds, chopped

- 1 teaspoon almond extract

- A pinch of sunflower seeds

- Stevia to taste

Directions:

1. Take a large bowl and pour coconut cream and coconut oil into it.

2. Whisk using an electric beater.

3. Whisk until the mixture becomes smooth and glossy.

4. Add cocoa powder slowly and mix well.

5. Add in the rest of the ingredients.

6. Pour into a bread pan lined with parchment paper.

7. Freeze until set.

8. Cut them into squares and serve.

Nutrition:

Total Carbs: 1g   Fiber: 1g Protein: 0g   Fat: 20g

Decisive Lime And Strawberry Popsicle

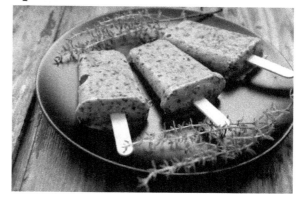

Preparation Time: 2 hours

Cooking Time: 0 minutes

Servings: 4

Ingredients:

- 1 tablespoon lime juice, fresh

- 1/4 cup strawberries, hulled and sliced

- 1/4 cup coconut almond milk, unsweetened and full fat

- 2 teaspoons natural sweetener

Directions:

1. Blend the listed ingredients in a blender until smooth.

2. Pour mix into popsicle molds and let them chill for 2 hours.

3. Serve and enjoy!

Nutrition:

Calories: 166

Fat: 17g

Carbohydrates: 3g

Protein: 1g

Ravaging Blueberry Muffin

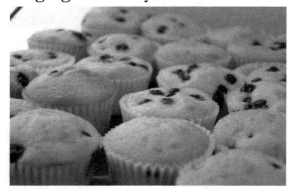

Preparation Time: 10 minutes

Cooking Time: 30 minutes

Servings: 4

Ingredients:

- 1 cup almond flour
- Pinch of sunflower seeds
- 1/8 teaspoon baking soda
- 1 whole egg
- 2 tablespoons coconut oil, melted
- 1/2 cup coconut almond milk
- 1/4 cup fresh blueberries

Directions:

1. Pre-heat your oven to 350 degrees F.

2. Line a muffin tin with paper muffin cups.

3. Add almond flour, sunflower seeds, baking soda to a bowl and mix, keep it on the side.

4. Take another bowl and add egg, coconut oil, coconut almond milk and mix.

5. Add mix to flour mix and gently combine until incorporated.

6. Mix in blueberries and fill the cupcakes tins with batter.

7. Bake for 20-25 minutes.

8. Enjoy!

Nutrition:

Calories: 167

Fat: 15g

Carbohydrates: 2.1g

Protein: 5.2g

CHAPTER 15:

Other Recipes

Baked Chicken

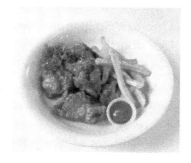

Preparation Time: 35 minutes

Cooking Time: 30 minutes

Servings: 4

Ingredients:

For the chicken:

- 4 chicken breasts, no bones or skins
- Two tsp. olive oil

For the seasoning:

- One-half tsp. black pepper
- One and one-half tbsp. brown sugar
- One tsp. thyme seasoning
- One tsp. paprika seasoning
- One-half tsp. salt
- One-fourth tsp. garlic powder
- For the garnish:
- One tbsp. parsley, chopped

Directions:

1. Heat the stove to the temperature of 425° Fahrenheit. Prepare a flat sheet with a rim with a layer of foil and set to the side. Blend the paprika, brown sugar, thyme, pepper, garlic powder, and salt in a glass dish until combined.
2. Arrange the chicken upside down on the prepped flat sheet and apply one tablespoon of the olive oil with a pastry brush. Dust with half of the mixed seasoning, covering completely and turn the chicken to the other side. Apply the remaining tablespoon of olive oil and the remaining seasoning making sure the chicken is completely covered. Heat for 18 minutes and remove from the stove.
3. Wait about 5 minutes before enjoying immediately.

Nutrition: Sodium: 403 mg Protein: 46 mg Fat: 7 mg Sugar: 4 mg Calories: 286

Cheesy Mushroom Risotto

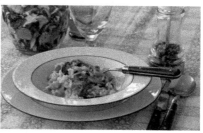

Preparation Time: 35 minutes

Cooking Time: 30 minutes

Servings: 4

Ingredients: One and three-fourths cups Swiss cheese, finely grated

- One medium onion, peeled and chopped

- Two tbsp. water
- Four and one-half cups vegetable broth, low-salt (See Helpful Tip below)
- Two tbsp. lemon juice
- One-fourth cup white wine - Two cups brown rice, uncooked
- One-third cup peas, thawed
- Two tbsp. olive oil, separated
- One-fourth tsp. black pepper
- One large leek, sliced thinly
- One and one-third cups mushrooms, sliced

Directions:

1. Remove the skin of the onion and chop into small chunks. Set to the side.
2. Wipe any excess dirt off of the mushrooms, slice and set aside.
3. Empty the vegetable broth into a deep pot and heat for approximately three minutes until it starts to bubble.
4. In the meantime, drizzle one tablespoon in a shallow skillet and brown the leeks, onion and two tablespoons of water for about two minutes.
5. Combine the rice, lemon juice, wine, and a cup of the vegetable stock.
6. Reduce while simmering for approximately 10 minutes until the water has completely evaporated.
7. Blend the mushrooms and add another cup of the vegetable stock, allowing reducing completely.
8. Keep adding a cup of vegetable stock as the water evaporates completely until it has been fully used. This will take about half an hour.
9. Finally, blend the Swiss cheese and peas to the stockpot and heat for another three minutes.
10. Serve immediately and enjoy!

Nutrition: Sodium: 123 mg Protein: 20 mg Fat: 8 mg Sugar: 5 mg Calories: 468

Chicken Gyros

Preparation Time: 15 minutes

Cooking Time: 10 minutes

Servings: 4

Ingredients:

- Two tbsp. lemon juice
- One tsp. cumin seasoning
- 4 pita bread slices
- One-half tsp. paprika seasoning
- One-fourth tsp. salt
- Two tsp. oregano seasoning
- One tsp. rosemary seasoning
- One-half cup onion, sliced
- 4 tbsp. olive oil
- One-half cup scallion, sliced
- Two cloves garlic, minced
- Two lb. chicken breast, no bones or skins
- One-fourth tsp. black pepper

Directions:

1. Prepare the onion by removing the outer skin and slicing along with the scallion. Set to the side.
2. Slice the chicken breast into small strips and transfer to a glass dish.
3. Heat a skillet on the burner.
4. Blend the paprika, cumin, lemon juice, salt, olive oil, and minced garlic in the dish with the chicken until integrated.
5. Finally, combine the oregano, rosemary, and pepper into the chicken dish.
6. Toss to ensure the chicken is evenly coated and transfer to the hot pan.
7. Heat for approximately 6 minutes while occasionally turning the meat to brown evenly.
8. Meanwhile, lay out the pita breads and top with the onions and green peppers.

9. Distribute the cooked chicken slices evenly on each of the pita breads.

10. Rotate the bread around the filling and enjoy immediately.

Nutrition: Sodium: 388 mg Protein: 4 mg Fat: 5 mg Sugar: 2 mg Calories: 159

Sun-Dried Tomato Basil Pizza

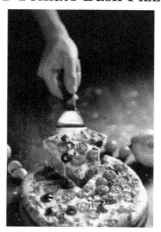

Preparation time: 30 minutes

Cooking time: 25 minutes

Servings: 4

Ingredients

- 12 inch prepared pizza crust purchased or made from mix…..1 crust
- Garlic cloves…..4
- Fat-free ricotta cheese…..1/2 cup
- Dry packed sun-dried tomatoes…..1/2 cup chopped
- Dried basil…..2 teaspoons
- Thyme…..1 teaspoon
- Red pepper flakes
- Parmesan cheese

Directions:

1. Preheat the oven to 475 °F (250 °C).
2. Lightly coat a 12-inch round pizza pie baking pan with cooking spray.
3. Sun-dried tomatoes need to be reconstituted before using. Place them in a bowl and pour boiled water over them until they are covered in water. Let stand for 5 minutes or until soft and pliable. Drain and chop.

4. Place the pizza crust in a round pizza pie-baking pan. Arrange garlic, cheese, and tomatoes on top of the pizza crust. Sprinkle basil and thyme evenly over the pizza.

5. Bake on the lowest rack of the oven until the pizza crust turns brown and the toppings are hot. About 20 minutes.

6. Cut the pizza into eight even slices and serve immediately.

7. Place the red-flaked pepper jar and the Parmesan jar out for individual use.

Nutrition: Total fat 2 g Calories 179 Protein 8 g Cholesterol 8 mg Total carbohydrate 32 g

Dietary fiber 2 g Monounsaturated fat 0.5 g Saturated fat trace Sodium 276 mg

White Sea Bass With Dill Relish

Preparation time: 15 minutes

Cooking time: 12 minutes

Servings: 4

Ingredients

- White Sea Bass fillets…..4 – 4 ounces each
- White onion…..1 1/2 tablespoons chopped
- Capers…..1 teaspoon drained
- Fresh dill…..1 1/2 teaspoons chopped
- Dijon mustard…..1 teaspoon
- Lemon juice…..1 teaspoon
- Lemon…..1 cut into quarters

Directions:

1. Preheat the oven to 375 °F (190 °C)

2. In a small bowl add the dill, capers, mustard, onion and lemon juice. Stir.

3. Place each fillet on a square of aluminum foil. Squeeze a lemon wedge over each fillet then spread 1/4 of the dill mixture over each piece of fish. Wrap the aluminum foil around the fish and bake or grill until the fish is opaque throughout. Cook 10 to 12 minutes. Serve.

Nutrition:

Total carbohydrate 3 g Dietary fiber 1 g

Sodium 129 mg Saturated fat < 0.5 g

Total fat 2 g Cholesterol 46 mg

Protein 21 g Monounsaturated fat < 0.5 g

Calories 119

Chinese Noodles With Spring Vegetables

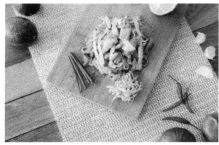

Preparation time: 20 minutes

Cooking time: 15 minutes

Servings: 4

Ingredients

- Chinese noodles......1 package (8 ounces)
- Fresh ginger.....1 tablespoon grated
- Garlic cloves.....2 finely chopped
- Reduced sodium soy sauce.....2 tablespoons
- Oyster sauce.....2 tablespoons
- Broccoli florets.....1 cup

- Bean sprouts.....1 cup
- Cherry tomatoes.....8 halved
- Fresh spinach.....1 cup chopped
- Scallions.....2 chopped
- Crushed red chili flakes (optional)
- Olive oil.....2 tablespoons

Directions:

1. Fill a large pot 3/4 full with water and bring to a boil. Add the Chinese noodles and cook until al dente, about 10 to 12 minutes. Drain the noodles. Set aside.

2. Heat the olive oil in a large frying pan over medium heat. Add ginger and garlic and cook until slightly brown. Add the soy sauce, oyster sauce and broccoli and stir for about 3 minutes. Add the remaining vegetables and stir until they are warm. Plate the noodles and top with the stir-fried vegetables. Add red chili flakes.

Nutrition: Total fat 9 g Calories 270 Protein 9 g Cholesterol 0 mg Total carbohydrate 38 g Dietary fiber 5 g Monounsaturated fat 4g Saturated fat 2 g Sodium 350 mg

Peanut Sauce Chicken Pasta

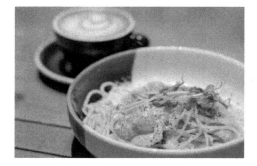

Preparation Time: 30 Minutes

Cooking Time: 30 Minutes

Servings: 4

Ingredients:

- 2 Teaspoons Olive Oil

- 6 Ounces Spaghetti, Whole Wheat
- 10 Ounces Snap Peas, Fresh & Trimmed & Sliced into Strips
- 2 Cups Carrots, Julienned
- 2 Cups Chicken, Cooked & Shredded
- 1 Cup Thai Peanut Sauce
- 1 Cucumber, Halved Lengthwise & Sliced Diagonally
- Cilantro, Fresh & Chopped

Directions:

1. Start by cooking spaghetti as the package instructs, and then drain them and rinse the noodles using cold water.
2. Heat your greased skillet using oil, placing it over medium heat.
3. Once it's hot, add in your snap peas and carrot. Cook for eight minutes, and stir in your spaghetti, chicken and peanut sauce. Toss well, and garnish with cucumber and cilantro.

Nutrition:

Calories: 403

Protein: 31 Grams

Fat: 15 Grams

Carbs: 43 Grams

Sodium: 432 mg

Cholesterol: 42 mg

Easy Barley Soup

Preparation Time: 30 Minutes

Cooking Time: 30 Minutes

Servings: 4

Ingredients:

- 1 Tablespoon Olive Oil
- 1 Onion, Chopped
- 5 Carrots, Chopped
- 2/3 Cup Barley, Quick Cooking

- 6 Cups Chicken Broth, Reduced Sodium
- 1/2 Teaspoon Black Pepper
- 2 Cups Baby Spinach, Fresh
- 2 Cups Turkey Breast, Cooked & Cubed

Directions:

1. Start by getting a saucepan and heat your oil over medium high heat.
2. Stir in your carrots and onion and sauté for five minutes before adding in your barley and broth. Bring it to a boil before reducing too low to simmer. Cook for fifteen minutes.
3. Stir in your pepper, spinach and turkey. Mix well before serving.

Nutrition:

Calories: 208 Protein: 21 Grams

Fat: 4 Grams Carbs: 23 Grams

Sodium: 662 mg Cholesterol: 37 mg

Curry Chicken Pockets

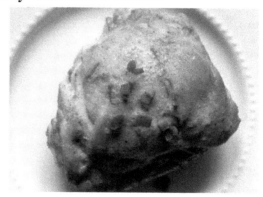

Preparation Time: 35 Minutes

Cooking Time: 35 Minutes

Servings: 4

Ingredients:

- 2 Cups Chicken, Cooked & Chopped
- 1/2 Cup Celery, Chopped
- 1/3 Cup Ricotta Cheese, Part Skim

- 1/ Cup Carrot, Shredded
- 1 Teaspoon Curry Powder
- 1 Tablespoon Apricot Preserved
- 10 Ounces Refrigerated Pizza Dough
- 1/4 Teaspoon Sea Salt
- 1/4 Teaspoon Ground Cinnamon

Directions:

1. Mix your carrot, ricotta, preserves, celery, chicken, cinnamon, salt and curry powder.
2. Spread the pizza dough and slice it into six equal squares.
3. Divide your mixture between each one, and then fold the corners of each towards the center and pinch them together. Put them on the baking sheet, baking at 375 for fifteen minutes. They should turn golden brown.
4. Allow them to cool before serving warm.

Nutrition:

Calories: 415 Protein: 31.2 Grams

Fat: 32.7 Grams Carbs: 14.7 Grams

Sodium: 277 mg

Cholesterol: 4.1 mg

Apple Swiss Panini

Preparation time: 10 minutes

Cooking time: 5 minutes

Servings: 4

Ingredients:

- 8 slices whole grain bread
- 1/4 cup nonfat honey mustard
- 2 crisp apples, sliced
- 6 ounces low fat Swiss cheese, thinly sliced
- 1 cup Arugula leaves
- Cooking spray

Directions:

1. Preheat Panini press on medium heat. If you don't have a Panini press, use a non-stick skillet.
2. Lightly spread honey mustard evenly on each slice of bread. Layer apple slices, cheese, and arugula leaves over 4 slices of bread.
3. Top each with remaining bread slices.
4. Lightly coat Panini press with cooking spray. Grill each sandwich for 3 to 5 minutes or until cheese has melted and bread has toasted.
5. Remove from pan and allow the Panini to cool slightly before serving.

Nutrition:

Calories 280 Total fat 4.5 g

Saturated fat 2 g Carbohydrate 44 g

Protein 17 g Fiber 5 g

Sodium 480 mg Potassium 288 mg

Magnesium 53 mg Calcium 458 mg

Heartfelt Tuna Melt

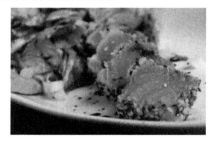

Preparation time: 5 minutes

Cooking time: 3 minutes

Servings: 4

Ingredients:

- 6 ounces white tuna packed in water, drained
- 1/3 cup chopped celery
- 1/4 cup chopped onion

- 1/4 cup low fat Russian salad dressing
- 2 whole-wheat English muffins
- 3 ounces reduced-fat Cheddar cheese, grated
- Salt and black pepper to taste

Directions:

1. Preheat broiler.
2. Combine tuna, celery, onion and salad dressing. Season with salt and pepper. Toast English muffin halves. Place split-side-up on baking sheet and top each with 1/4 of tuna mixture. Broil for 2-3 minutes or until heated through.
3. Top with cheese.

Nutrition:

Calories 210 Total fat 6 g

Saturated fat 3 g Carbohydrates 20 g

Protein 19 g Fiber 3 g

Sodium 417 mg Potassium 157 mg

Magnesium 17 mg Calcium 185 mg

- 3 tablespoons plain fat free yogurt
- 1 tablespoon lemon juice
- 2 tablespoons red bell pepper
- 1 tablespoon red onion
- 1 teaspoon capers, rinsed and chopped
- Pinch of dill, fresh or dried
- Black pepper to taste
- 3 lettuce leaves
- 3 pieces small whole wheat pita bread

Directions:

1. Mix first 8 ingredients together in a small bowl to make a salmon salad. Place 1 lettuce leaf and 1/3 cup salmon salad inside each pita.

Nutrition:

180 calories 4 g total fat

0.5 g saturated fat 19 g carbohydrates

19 g protein 3 g fiber 420 mg sodium

331 mg potassium 43 mg magnesium

60 mg calcium

Salmon Salad

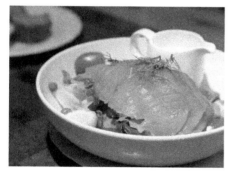

Preparation time: 10 minutes

Cooking time: 0 minutes

Servings: 3

Ingredients:

- 3/4 cup canned Alaskan salmon

Mayo-Less Tuna Salad

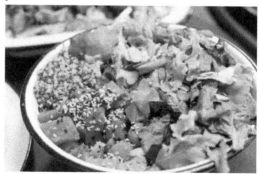

Preparation time: 10 minutes

Cooking time: 0 minutes

Serving: 2

Ingredients:

- 5 Ounces tuna, canned in water, drained

- 1 Cup cooked pasta
- 1 Tablespoon extra-virgin olive oil
- 1 Tablespoon red wine vinegar
- 1/4 Cup green onion, sliced
- 2 Cups arugula
- 1 Tablespoon Parmesan cheese, shredded
- 1/2 Teaspoon black pepper

Directions:

2. In a large bowl, toss tuna with vinegar, arugula, oil, onion, and cooked pasta.
3. Divide the dish between 2 plates equally.
4. Top with pepper and Parmesan before serving.
5. Serve hot.

Nutrition:

Calories: 84

Total Fat: 7.9 g

Saturated Fat: 1.5 g

Total Carbs: 2.4 g

Dietary Fiber: 0.8 g

Total Sugars: 0.7 g

Cholesterol: 2 mg

Sodium: 51 mg

Protein: 2 g

Calcium: 75 mg

Iron: 1 mg

Potassium: 125 mg

Vitamin D: 0 mcg

28 Day-Meal Plan

Day	Breakfast	Lunch	Dinner	Snacks
1	Sweet Potatoes With Coconut Flakes	Corn And Beans Tortillas	Cod Tacos	Egg Rolls In A Bowl
2	Flaxseed & Banana Smoothie	Chicken And Spinach Mix	Zucchini Fritters	Instant Pot Quinoa
3	Fruity Tofu Smoothie	Garlic Chickpeas Fritters	Chickpeas Stew	Pork Beef Bean Nachos
4	French Toast With Applesauce	Cheddar Cauliflower Bowls	Lemon Chicken Salad	Pressure Cooker Cranberry Hot Wings
5	Banana-Peanut Butter 'N Greens Smoothie	Salmon Salad	Asparagus Salad	Bacon Hot Dog Bites
6	Baking Powder Biscuits	Chicken And Tomato Mix	Tomato Beef Stew	Instant Pot Cocktail Wieners
7	Oatmeal Banana Pancakes With Walnuts	Salmon And Olives Salad	Rosemary Pork Chops	Pressure Cooker Braised Pulled Ham
8	Creamy Oats, Greens & Blueberry Smoothie	Shrimp Salad	Balsamic Shrimp Salad	Mini Teriyaki Turkey Sandwiches
9	Banana & Cinnamon Oatmeal	Turkey Tortillas	Eggplant And Tomato Stew	Hoisin Meatballs
10	Bagels Made Healthy	Parsley Green Beans Soup	Beef And Scallions Mix	Cuban Pulled Pork Sandwiches
11	Cereal With Cranberry-Orange Twist	Beef Skillet	Lime Turkey Stew	Instant Pot Polenta
12	No Cook Overnight Oats	Thyme Beef And Tomatoes	Beef And Beans Salad	Asian Glazed Meatballs
13	Avocado Cup With Egg	Pork Soup	Squash And Peppers Stew	Jalapeno Cheddar Cornbread
14	Mediterranean Toast	Shrimp And Spinach Salad	Beef And Cabbage Stew	Egg Rolls In A Bowl

15	Sweet Potatoes With Coconut Flakes	Raspberry Shrimp And Tomato Salad	Pork Stew	Instant Pot Quinoa
16	Flaxseed & Banana Smoothie	Corn And Beans Tortillas	Cod Tacos	Pork Beef Bean Nachos
17	Fruity Tofu Smoothie	Chicken And Spinach Mix	Zucchini Fritters	Pressure Cooker Cranberry Hot Wings
18	French Toast With Applesauce	Garlic Chickpeas Fritters	Chickpeas Stew	Bacon Hot Dog Bites
19	Banana-Peanut Butter 'N Greens Smoothie	Cheddar Cauliflower Bowls	Lemon Chicken Salad	Instant Pot Cocktail Wieners
20	Baking Powder Biscuits	Salmon Salad	Asparagus Salad	Pressure Cooker Braised Pulled Ham
21	Oatmeal Banana Pancakes With Walnuts	Chicken And Tomato Mix	Tomato Beef Stew	Mini Teriyaki Turkey Sandwiches
22	Creamy Oats, Greens & Blueberry Smoothie	Salmon And Olives Salad	Rosemary Pork Chops	Hoisin Meatballs
23	Banana & Cinnamon Oatmeal	Shrimp Salad	Balsamic Shrimp Salad	Cuban Pulled Pork Sandwiches
24	Bagels Made Healthy	Turkey Tortillas	Eggplant And Tomato Stew	Instant Pot Polenta
25	Cereal With Cranberry-Orange Twist	Parsley Green Beans Soup	Beef And Scallions Mix	Asian Glazed Meatballs
26	No Cook Overnight Oats	Beef Skillet	Lime Turkey Stew	Jalapeno Cheddar Cornbread
27	Avocado Cup With Egg	Thyme Beef And Tomatoes	Beef And Beans Salad	Smoked Salad
28	Mediterranean Toast	Pork Soup	Squash And Peppers Stew	Mesmerizing Avocado And Chocolate Pudding

Conversion Tables

Volume Equivalents (Liquid)

US STANDARD	US STANDARD (OUNCES)	METRIC (APPROXIMATE)
2 tablespoons	1 fl. oz.	30 mL
1/4 cup	2 fl. oz.	60 mL
1/2 cup	4 fl. oz.	120 mL
1 cup	8 fl. oz.	240 mL
11/2 cups	12 fl. oz.	355 mL
2 cups or 1 pint	16 fl. oz.	475 mL
4 cups or 1 quart	32 fl. oz.	1 L
1 gallon	128 fl. oz.	4 L

Volume Equivalents (Dry)

US STANDARD	METRIC (APPROXIMATE)
1/4 teaspoon	1 mL
1/2 teaspoon	2 mL
1 teaspoon	5 mL
1 tablespoon	15 mL
1/4 cup	59 mL
cup	79 mL
1/2 cup	118 mL
1 cup	177 mL

Oven Temperatures

FAHRENHEIT (F)	CELSIUS (C) (APPROXIMATE)
250°F	120 °C
300°F	150°C
325°F	165°C
350°F	180°C
375°F	190°C
400°F	200°C
425°F	220°C
450°F	230°C

Weight Equivalents

US STANDARD	METRIC (APPROXIMATE)
1/2 ounce	15 g
1 ounce	30 g
2 ounces	60 g
4 ounces	115 g
8 ounces	225 g
12 ounces	340 g
16 ounces or 1 pound	455 g

Recipe Index

T

V

W

Z

Conclusion

Thank you for making it to the end. Initially, when the DASH diet was created, it was solely created to reduce and stop the spread of hypertension, but it was later discovered that people who adopted the DASH diet were able to lose their weight to a considerable and moderate level. The reason for this was because of what the DASH diet entails that has made it effective for weight loss. As we end this book, here are some tips on how you can make your DASH diet work:

Remove processed and junk food from your refrigerator: With the DASH diet, it is required that processed and junk food is rid of in the refrigerator because this food contains a high level of calories and unhealthy fats. Replace the processed and junk foods with fresh fruits, vegetables, grains, and raw nuts. Throwing away the junks may seem too much to do; however, the best thing to do is refraining from buying them.

Prepare a grocery list: Before heading to the supermarket, ensure you have a list of the DASH diet food list to purchase. This is to help to refrain from what is not on the grocery list in respect to the DASH diet

Prepare your meal whenever possible: No matter how sweet and healthy a meal prepared in the restaurant is, you don't know the combination of the ingredients, whether it is a detriment to your weight loss or not. It is therefore important to ensure you prepare your meal all by yourself most times and by so doing you can monitor what goes into your body regarding the DASH diet

Stock your kitchen with DASH food: To avoid the temptation of eating foods that are detrimental to your weight loss, stock your kitchen with DASH food from time to time. By so doing, you get accustomed to the DASH diet

Avoid eating unhealthy snacks: Do away with snacks with unhealthy seasonings rather than go for snacks like popcorn cooked in olive oil and seasoned with garlic.

Consume less sodium: Food like bread, baked food, breakfast cereals, condiments, sauce, and canned products contain a high level of sodium, and these must be taken the required level to avoid posing a danger to the bodyweight.

Checking of labels: Most people are victims of the act of not checking labels on food items purchased; thus, endangering their health. Check the labels of every food item in your kitchen and refrigerator and dispose of anything that has a high intake of sodium, sugar, white flour, saturated or trans fats.

Portion control and serving sizes: This involves eating a variety of food in the right proportion and getting the required amount of nutrients needed. Eating to get overfed is what most people do all for the sake of eating to one's satisfaction, with this simple act, most people don't know that obesity can be gotten this, thus with the DASH diet, individuals know the amount of food to be taken with regards to the normal body functioning system and thereby having a balanced body weight.

Avoid Sedentary habit: This is a lifestyle that involves little or no physical activities. Examples of sedentary lifestyles are sitting with the computer all day long, reading all day long, or watching television most hours of the day. This kind of habit is not encouraged in the DASH diet, thereby not leading to unnecessary weight gain—more of a reason why the DASH diet encourages physical exercises.

I hope you have learned something!

A Short message from the Author:

Hey, are you enjoying the book? I'd love to hear your thoughts!
Many readers do not know how hard reviews are to come by, and how much they help an author.

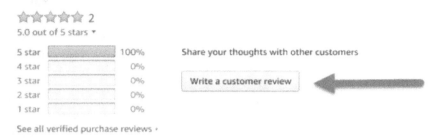

I would be incredibly thankful if you could take just 60 seconds to write a brief review on Amazon, even if it's just a few sentences!

If you have purchased the paperback version, just going to your purchases section in Amazon or search this book through Amazon (Title and Name of the Author) and Click "Write a Review".

Thank you for taking the time to share your thoughts!
Your review will genuinely make a difference for me and help gain exposure for my work.

Victoria Wills

CPSIA information can be obtained
at www.ICGtesting.com
Printed in the USA
LVHW100320180121
676770LV00013B/398